W0113170

Brief Narrative Practice in Single-Session Therapy

Brief Narrative Practice in Single-Session Therapy emphasizes collaboration, meaning making, and relational ethics in single-session conversations. Chapters provide a thorough orientation to the therapy and address the diverse circumstances clinicians face in these conversations.

Separating from many long-held traditions in therapy, this book explores a guiding framework and the accompanying micro-skills that therapeutic conversations demand. In these pages, readers will learn how to recalibrate their listening habits and talk differently about problems in ways that help them quickly hear and generate possibilities.

All those who provide psychotherapy, counselling, and coaching in time-constrained contexts will find this book useful and engaging, including those working in crisis and call-in settings, walk-in clinics, medical centres, and live-in contexts where change conversations are brief.

Scot J. Cooper is a registered psychotherapist and manager for child and youth mental health services in Ontario, Canada. With over 25 years of practice and teaching, Scot is one of the key voices shaping the quick access mental health service landscape in Canada.

Brief Narrative Practice in Single-Session Therapy

Scot J. Cooper

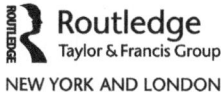
Routledge
Taylor & Francis Group

NEW YORK AND LONDON

Cover image: BlackJack3D © Getty Images.

First published 2024
by Routledge
605 Third Avenue, New York, NY 10158

and by Routledge
4 Park Square, Milton Park, Abingdon, Oxon, OX14 4RN

Routledge is an imprint of the Taylor & Francis Group, an informa business

Library of Congress Cataloging-in-Publication Data
Names: Cooper, Scot J., author.
Title: Brief narrative practice in single-session therapy / Scot J. Cooper.
Identifiers: LCCN 2023047305 (print) | LCCN 2023047306 (ebook) |
ISBN 9781032556208 (hbk) | ISBN 9781032556192 (pbk) |
ISBN 9781003431688 (ebk)
Subjects: LCSH: Single-session psychotherapy. |
Narrative therapy. | Single-session psychotherapy–Methodology. |
Narrative therapy–Methodology.
Classification: LCC RC480.55 .C673 2024 (print) |
LCC RC480.55 (ebook) | DDC 616.89/165–dc23/eng/20231227
LC record available at https://lccn.loc.gov/2023047305
LC ebook record available at https://lccn.loc.gov/2023047306

ISBN: 9781032556208 (hbk)
ISBN: 9781032556192 (pbk)
ISBN: 9781003431688 (ebk)

DOI: 10.4324/9781003431688

Typeset in Times New Roman
by Newgen Publishing UK

Contents

Acknowledgments

A great deal of the writing and work reflected within this book took place on or near the unceded land of the Anishinaabe, Haudenosaunee, and Attawandaron Nations. As a white person of settler background, I acknowledge that I have access to this land because of colonial violence that is not solely historic but continues today and is deeply intertwined with all inequities. Our agreement for this territory is reflected in the Two Row Wampum Belt. The Two Row is a living treaty that holds each nation to living in peace and friendship with non-interference forever; as long as the grass is green, as long as the water runs downhill, as long as the sun rises in the East and sets in the West, and as long as our Mother Earth will last.

In the same way that I am sensitive to my place here on the land and how that came to be, I am sensitive to how my voice becomes centred within this book. This is especially present for me when I facilitate workshops on the material, as many have contributed to what I am sharing. Given this, foremost I wish to express gratitude to the people and families that I have been fortunate to meet with over many years. You have taught me a great deal through your generosity in sharing your experiences and contributing to this book.

Over the years, I have had very skilled teachers. The first workshop I ever attended was at Brief Therapy Training Centres International™ (BTTC-I) in Toronto, Ontario and led by Scott Miller, Ph.D. I was hooked immediately, and that workshop set me on the path I have been following for several decades now. This was not necessarily because of how talented of a presenter Scott is, and for those who have seen Scott present, you know he is tremendous, but because of the respectful approach he was sharing. I can still recall the video he showed where the outcome was in a man deciding on his own to attend the hospital where he would be safe as opposed to authorities enforcing his confinement.

I've been most influenced by Jim Duvall, who founded BTTC-I and took me in as an adjunct faculty. He, along with Eric King, shaped the 'Brief' presence in Ontario and throughout Canada. Gratitude for all you have done. Thanks to Kevin Clouthier, who was the first to introduce me to single session therapy, again at BTTC-I. He shattered a glass ceiling to what might be possible within significant time constraint. I also want to express gratitude to Yvonne Dolan, who I was talking with after one of her workshops on solution-focused brief therapy in 2001. As a parting comment, she asked me, "So, when is your book coming out?" She knew I was new to the field, and she had this look in her eye like she was up to something. That comment has always stayed with me as I guess Yvonne had intended, and perhaps it has sprouted this many years later. That simple question suggested to me it might be a possibility one day. Yvonne is another fantastic SFBT trainer with a background in hypnotherapy.

I miss Michael White, the co-founder of narrative therapy, as I am sure most do who had crossed paths with him. There is not another library of ideas and work that has had a more profound influence on my practice. I have done my best to honour the quality of his contribution and continue to keep these practices alive in a field overridden with stock approaches and practices of diagnosis. I knew Michael a bit as we spent time together with the Neighbouring Communities Project in 2007. This was a relationship building initiative between the people of Six Nations of the Grand River and the people of Caledonia who had come into conflict related to a longstanding land rights dispute. Michael generously found time to come to lead the community assignment, and we stayed in contact through to his passing. It was through Michael that I came connected to the narrative family. Thanks as well to Maggie Carey and Shona Russell for staying connected and answering my questions.

Finally, through this career, I have seen my twins Ben and Grace grow to become young adults and Monica and I couldn't be prouder of them. I hope one day they can find a field they enjoy as much as I have in meeting with children, youth, and families to address distress.

Note to Readers

As any practice is located in shifting time, clinical standards, and culture, there is no perfect therapeutic approach. Given this, no approach or recommendation is guaranteed to be safe or effective in all circumstances. This volume provides material for the exploration of theory and a corresponding skills-set for professionals practicing in psychotherapy and mental health. It is to accompany training, apprenticeship and practice, and for discussion in peer review and/or clinical supervision, which is an important part of clinical practice.

Privacy note: Identifying information, contexts, and names have been altered to ensure privacy. Stories and vignettes shared, unless otherwise stated, are composite accounts. Any association to a personal account would be happenstance. As conversations are shaped by conversation maps, similarities in content are common. Thank you to those who have granted permission for their stories to be shared and for their contribution to our learning.

Introduction

Brevity does not necessarily mean superficial; the right haiku can be much more to the point and soul stirring than a long, plodding novel–or therapy.

(Hoyt, 2021, p. 68)

You might have experienced this too, reflecting back over life I can recall a handful of conversations that have stayed with me in some way. These may not have been long winded, or particularity sought out, yet they were meaningful at the time and helped to shape my life in important ways. Like throwing a rock into a flowing river, the river doesn't flow the same afterwards. Other metaphors apply. These conversations can be like tipping the first domino or beginning to role a snowball down a hill. They set things in motion. I believe we all have had these kinds of conversations at one time or another. They involve the kind of talk that requires you to think differently about yourself or reveals unforeseen ways forward in difficult times. These are conversations that shake how you knew the world or ideas you had settled into. However, what this tells us is that these kinds of experiences are possible. A single conversation can touch a life in a way that is significant. It can ripple and reverberate through the years.

Michael Hoyt, one of the lead innovators of single session therapy reminds us of this with the above quote. A single session, when timely, skillfully executed, and fitting, can take people to places in meaning making that they could not have arrived at on their own. Like the right haiku, communication is focused and efficient, spawning brevity. That has been the influence of the brief therapies that has rippled through to today making way for the emergence of single session therapy as part of diverse service menu.

Single session therapy (SST) finds its roots stretching back to the brief therapies in the 1950s when Don Jackson founded the Mental Research Institute (MRI) in Palo Alto, California. The importance of that development in psychotherapy today cannot be overstated. MRI was an institute for the study of family interactions and the teaching of family therapy. The MRI 'Brief Therapy Centre'

DOI: 10.4324/9781003431688-1

was one of the projects at MRI. Within an atmosphere of innovation, they sought to focus on how to make therapy more effective and efficient (Watzlawick, Weakland & Fisch, 1974). It brought together many rigorous thinkers and researchers. Mavericks at the time, the group included influence from Gregory Bateson, consultation with Psychiatrist Milton Erickson, and contributions from Richard Fisch, Jay Haley, Jules Riskin, Virginia Satir, Paul Watzlawick, and John Weakland.

They drew from eclectic schools of thought, including communication theory, anthropology, ecology, psychiatry, and social work. The emphasis was on seeking what they could do to get people to address their own difficulties rather than promoting insight. This shift to the Interactional approach focused on patterns of family interaction, and the family's view of the problem. Those times introduced systemic thinking; looking for pattern, difference, with attention to process and relationship.

The development of brief therapy challenged many long held and widely accepted structures and practices of psychotherapy. It represented a significant departure from the individual intra-psychic methods that dominated the time, such as psychoanalytic work. During a time when people were seen for years through hundreds of sessions, Brief therapy embraced brevity. That brevity was not about doing the popular therapy of the time in fewer sessions. Rather, brevity came about as a consequence of a new way of conceptualizing human problems and ensuing ideas about how to address psychiatric problems (Weakland et al., 1977). With the focus on how to make therapy more effective, it began a move away from understanding people through a biomedical lens towards a non-pathologizing approach locating problems as outside of people. Drawing from Erikson's work, the idea of utilization meant working with what people had to offer, what they brought with them to the session in terms of meanings, experiences, and actions. An understanding of the importance and use of language as shaping people's meanings or realities emerged. It involved a look at relationships and context of people's lives, and the understanding that people could intervene in their lives to make change. This reflected a belief in people. We can see these early shifts as threading together the constellation of therapies under the brief umbrella that emerged in the decades that followed.

This early work at MRI seeded something special, shaping what I call the contemporary brief therapies. The stories of development at MRI portray an atmosphere of abundant curiosity, rigour of study, investigation, and research. The group had studied communication in diverse ways, observing how to train a guide dog to how a ventriloquist communicated with their dummy. They observed animals in the zoo and later focused on the communication of those described as schizophrenics. Listening to the early recordings of the Bateson

Group after returning from observing Milton Erickson, you can hear the enthusiasm as they wrestled with what they had seen, wringing out of the confusion new ideas, attempting to discern what was useful and efficient in therapeutic encounters. They used audio and film recordings much like a modern sports team would nowadays. They reviewed their work over and over, discussed it with colleagues from different vantage points, watched each other work from behind a mirror, and implemented new ideas and reviewed some more. Untethering from what was commonplace seemed to set in motion an ethos of a sort that I believe still ripples through the brief therapies and made possible the emergence of single session therapy.

Moving into the 1980s, innovation continued to spark from connections to the MRI Brief Therapy Team as Steve de Shazer, trained by John Weakland, co-developed solution-focused brief therapy, alongside his partner Insoo Kim Berg. Emerging through the late 1980s and 1990s Steve, Insoo and colleagues at the Brief Family Therapy Centre in Milwaukee would meet with people in their basement with colleagues sitting on the stairs watching and learning. What they were crafting ushered in one of the most exciting shifts in the field as an approach to change emerged based around building possibility from what people already know to do to shape a preferred future. This involved a move away from talking about and detailing problems towards a focus on exceptions to when problems were happening and detailing the life people would prefer to be living. This was a time when meta-theory was changing, and the brief genre embraced post-modernism, social-constructionism, post-structuralism and feminist theory.

Around the same time, Michael White from Australia with early interest in many of Bateson's ideas, began collaborating with David Epston from New Zealand crafting narrative therapy (White & Epston, 1990). This is a therapy shaped by the text analogy or story, informed by post-structural and feminist ideas as well as thinking from diverse fields such as anthropology, ethnography, and philosophy. With an ethos in harmony with the early work of MRI Group, Michael and David embarked on what can be described as a journey of exploration to new and unexplored places in therapeutic conversations. Michael called for a re-visioning of the therapeutic context and the dismantling of long accepted structures and practices (White, 2011, p. 45). He and David would come to introduce the practices of externalizing conversations, re-authoring, re-membering conversations, and unique uses of documenting (White & Epston, 1990). They would bring into focus attention to power relations and the relational ethics of practice, considering the possible effects of what we do on shaping people's lives and the ways they come to see themselves. Their contribution to the field is extremely rich in theory and practice.

As part of his training intensives, Michael often did live demonstrations of his practice with children, adults, and families. This was a rare practice in the field. I had only ever seen Insoo do something similar. Many of those meetings have been video recorded and are part of a large library of his work housed at the Dulwich Centre in Adelaide. It was in this tradition practiced by Michael that we could tease out a brief narrative approach. He showed what was possible within a single conversation. Michael himself was confident about the usefulness of those training session demonstrations. I remember driving from the airport in 2010[1] and talking with him about what could be accomplished within the time constraint of a single session. He had noted how far together therapist and participant could travel from the known and familiar in one conversation. We speculated about what we were learning about ways to extend the influence of conversation well beyond the conversation itself. This is a legacy Michael has left us. We are able to discern from those recordings brief narrative practices relevant to time constrained therapeutic contexts.

I came to these brief therapies through my time at Brief Therapy Training Centres International™ (BTTC-I) in Toronto, Ontario, under the leadership of Jim Duvall and Eric King. As a graduate of the brief therapy extern program, I joined the training team from 2000 through to 2012. Karen Young, a skilled trainer and narrative therapist, later also joined as we immersed further into narrative influenced work. Those were exciting times. Jim [2] had seemed to foster some of that MRI/SFBT/Narrative atmosphere of excitement for what might be possible in therapeutic conversations. There was a spirit of exploration and discovery, connecting with like-minded people, discussing the practices at gatherings as we sought to stretch our practice. The Institute had hosted several conferences and trainings connected to the extern program that brought the innovators such as Richard Fisch, Steve and Insoo, Michael and David to Toronto. There was a stream of post-modern trainers including Yvonne Dolan, Jill Freedom, Tom Lund, Joe Eron, Scott Miller, Eve Lipchik, Ron Krawl, John Walter, and Heather Fiske. Jim and the Institute certainly shaped the landscape in Ontario, keeping alive these ideas spawn from the 1950s and refined through the decades since.

As I mentioned, it was in late 1997 that I was first introduced to single session therapy at a workshop by Kevin Clouthier hosted by BTTC-I. He was experimenting with several concepts and practices back then, such as the notion of bi-furcation and questions from competency-focused therapies in an emerging post-modern therapeutic context. Kevin planted the notion that much more was possible in my conversations with people, despite how brief they sometimes were. The Institute had been offering single sessions as part of the extern program as a teaching device, so the idea of specific single session therapy made sense. Visiting trainers would facilitate a session for the externs to watch and learn from and, as I mentioned, Michael offered live demonstration as part of training intensives.

In 1998, I joined a growing rural agency to meet with children and families but also to bring my teachings about brief practice to life at the agency. Again, how fortunate I was to find myself where the atmosphere of exploration and discovery was encouraged. In 2002 we began call ahead single session consultations, eventually moving to a full walk-in clinic in 2006 providing service to children and their families modelled after what Karen Young had been doing since 2002 at a similar agency in Burlington. However, this derivative of service delivery was part of a larger movement in Ontario that saw the proliferation of single session/walk-in clinic therapy throughout the province.

It can be said that current single session practice is young and growing. There is more to be discovered in terms of how to be most useful to people seeking service. In reflection, the influence of those early MRI days, its ethos perhaps still shapes the spirit within which we continue to grow therapeutic practice relevant to single session and/or walk-in therapy contexts. Old ideas are unsettled, and new ideas are explored and practiced. I believe we have turned the corner on the skepticism that would often greet us in training forums. There is a population in the field that recognizes how quick access SST is an important and ethical part of a diverse service menu.

Many stories have sustained me in my exploration of single session practice and assured me of the difference these conversations can make to the lives of young people. For instance, Jacob, a 10-year-old, made visible the future 'bullying' wanted for him; that of an extinguished life. Hearing Jacob declare his 'humanitarian beliefs' and what it took to live these beliefs in the face of such assault was inspiring. To see his relief as 'bullying' came out of the shadows and counter-steps were revealed, along with allies for safety, was a great distance to travel in one talk. Or perhaps a gift to me was to learn from Bill how his dear friend who had tragically died had talked him out of his plan to massacre his classmates, who had verbally and physically tormented him. He took advice from his friend and their friendship became Bill's reason to live and to resist coaching from peers to end his life. Bill's continued life remains a tribute to his past friend who would have been proud to know he embraced a safe life and had moved to live with his father, free from the harassment of a past peer group. Stories like Bill's emphasize the importance of quick access to therapeutic conversations where new meanings can be forged and safety shored up. I still remember

Vanessa's discovery that she is not 'crazy' despite her given diagnosis of attention deficit disorder and learning disabilities. As it turned out, her self-proclaimed 'randomness' had the special ability to bring humour and fun to her relationships. And in fact, she was employing several skills, including focus, interest, and a commitment to her learning. As this alternate territory of identity emerged, what fun it was to see Vanessa counter the claims made about her by professionals.

It's through a brief narrative approach that these conversations are made possible. With this book, my aim is to share what might be possible with you by providing a window into a brief narrative practice at a single session therapy walk-in clinic. I hope you find ideas and inspiration for your own practice and embark on a useful journey of exploration and growth.

Chapter 1 reviews the therapeutic landscape in which single session therapy has emerged and grown throughout Ontario. I start there because of the important influence the work in Ontario has made for several decades. Chapters 2 and 3 outline the mind-set favourable to brief narrative conversations and a revision of the therapeutic context. This is a move away from traditional psychological frames to the 'rite of passage' metaphor, where change is understood as movement in life. This revised concept shapes how we hear people's expression of distress and opens a range of possibilities for therapeutic conversations. Chapter 4 details the listening that comes from an understanding that any expression is radically plural.

Proceeding Chapters 5 through 7 will detail the micro skills that accompany the phases of a single session conversation. While the metaphor may seem like a simplification, attention to each of these phases highlights the practice nuances that forge a complete therapy.

Chapters 8 and 9 share documenting practices relevant to SST. Narrative therapy has a long history of using documentation to extend the influence of the conversation and to recruit and audience to change. These chapters share the practice of collaborative or concurrent documentation within the single session and many relevant uses of documentation. This practice sets SST apart from more traditional approaches.

Externalizing conversations is the focus of Chapter 10, reviewing White's externalizing conversations, maps and application to time constraint conversations. That sets the stage for Chapter 11 giving specific attention to the co-authoring of counter-stories. These are specific stories that set out to address negative identity claims. The practice vignette includes another sample of a take-away document.

Within Chapter 12 I share some of the important conversational options emerging from narrative therapy and elsewhere relevant to addressing the effects of trauma in a single session. Trauma is a loaded word with many meanings in contemporary culture. Escaping the dominant discourse of trauma opens many possibilities for these conversations to make a difference. Many of the practices are brought to life with a vignette in Chapter 13 as a young person devises their 'game plan for their life' to escape abuse and neglect.

Chapters 14 through 16 take a closer look at special topics, including options for addressing loss, re-conceptualizing the experience of crisis and options to assist practitioners and children to navigate the politics of separation/divorce at the walk-in.

Chapter 17 explores the development of concepts for living in SST through the use of activities with children and families. My intention is to share what's possible moving away from verbal exchange into activity and body awareness. Finally, Chapter 18 presents a post session measure of process and outcome for SST. This chapter directs attention to how 'what we look to measure' also shapes 'how we do what we do' in practice. A feedback tool is offered to elicit feedback following a single session to ensure our practices are in harmony with brief narrative, relational ethics.

Moving forward, let's first travel to the evolving therapeutic landscape to set the scene for the exploration ahead.

Notes

1 Following the Neighbouring Communities community initiative in 2007, Michael generously made time to re-visit the communities to provide follow-up consultation. He was excited about the Pen Pal Project, an initiative started by community member Suzie Miller that found support through the community gathering in 2007. See www. penpalproject.ca for an archive of the project.
2 For the history of the BTTC-I and to learn about Jim's vision, which at the heart, looked to establish affiliations and collaborations see Duvall (1994). Speaking to an ethos of sort, he notes, "…we believe in a unifying and inclusive approach to brief therapy and, in fact, view it more as an overarching philosophy that includes constantly evolving emphasis and contributions, than any particular "model". We also believe that the work is more powerful, interesting and a lot more fun when we form collaborative and cooperative relationships with our colleagues" (p. 77).

References

Hoyt, M. F. (2021). The hope and joy of single session thinking and practice. In M. F. Hoyt, J. Young, & P. Rycroft (Eds.), *Single-session thinking and practice in global, cultural, and familial contexts: Expanding applications* (pp. 29–41). Routledge.

Watzlawick, P., Weakland, J. H., & Fisch, R. (1974). *Change: Principles of problem formation and problem resolution.* New York: Norton.

Weakland, J., Fisch, R., Watzlawick, P., & Bodin, A. M. (1977). Brief therapy: Focused problem resolution. In *The interactional view: Studies at the Mental Research Institute Palo Alto 1965–1974* (pp. 274–299). W. W. Norton and Company.

White, M. (2011). *Narrative practice: Continuing the conversations*. W.W. Norton, New York.

White, M. & Epston, D. (1990). *Narrative means to therapeutic ends*. New York: W.W. Norton.

Chapter 1

The Therapeutic Landscape

For a very long time, wait times have plagued mental health services. Many of the very organizational structures themselves, for instance, in children's mental health, are designed for waitlist models of service delivery. Capacity is devoted to monitoring waitlists, and accreditation standards are in place for waitlist oversight, all of which, to me, fosters a general complacency with the idea that those who are in distress can wait. Children in Ontario, Canada in 2020 experienced wait for service an average of 67 days with the longest waits up to two-and-a-half years for counselling and therapy (CMHO 2020 Report: Kids Can't Wait). However, with the emergence of walk-in and single session access, those who don't want to wait can access a complete session of psychotherapy in their time of need. This service innovation has emerged as an ethical part of a diverse service menu and is re-shaping the service landscape.

Single Session Therapy

As mentioned, the movement to work within time constraint had roots in the 1950s at MRI as efficient and effective therapies had been in development. The seminal book *Single Session Therapy: maximizing the effect of the first (and often only) therapeutic encounter* by Moshe Talmon (1990) outlined the practice of single session therapy and accompanying supporting research. It is infused with the traditions of the MRI brief therapy, solution-focused brief therapy, and others who had been working within specific time constraint. The past three decades have seen several important contributors defining the practice of single session therapy, each with their own nuances yet joined by common understandings about therapy, people, problems, and change (Talmon, 1990; Young, 2006; Slive & Bobele, 2011; Hoyt & Talmon, 2014; Dryden, 2019; Cannistra & Piccirilli, 2021).

Single session therapy (SST), as I know it on the Canadian landscape, provides a time to assist people to address their distress through collaboration, exploration, and discovery. Let me be clear that it is not triage; that is, readying people for an ongoing service. It does not involve a traditional genre of assessment

DOI: 10.4324/9781003431688-2

trying to detail the problem in order to prescribe treatment. It is not a time to point out positives or cheerlead[1] people to carry on through hard times. It is not a space for diagnosis.

SST is a complete therapy process and involves generative conversations with people seeking and building upon their knowledge and experience. People bring with them to these conversations a wealth of experience represented as concepts such as hopes for their life, treasured values, important beliefs, positive intentions, skills for living, abilities, commitments to valued principles, competencies, resiliencies, moral codes, and nourishing relationships that shape their expressions of life and can be utilized to live a preferred life. As well, people have taken initiative in their lives to address their problematic circumstances, which show up as exceptions to problems, unique outcomes, times when the problem was less intense or not around. All this material is available across the entire timeline to be canvassed and put to agentive use to address what they deem as distressing. We want to learn as much as we can from them, inviting them to mentor us in their experience, writing their ideas in quotes, co-creating plans of action, and referencing that material in take-away documents for future consultation.

Our contribution as the senior partner in the process is to facilitate a useful conversation, drawing primarily upon participants' ideas and experience, at times sharing what we bring to the process, such as our learning from other families, our education, and experience. Together, we co-develop plans of action or small next steps that fit into their world and culture. We invite practice and experimentation with these plans that may need fine tuning. Single session therapy is hard work and requires rigorous practice and reflection by the therapist.

The context in which the therapy takes place shapes the length of these conversations. At my clinic, we take a generous approach to time, noting it takes as long as it takes. Working with children and youth may require time well spent meeting them through stories of their competence as a means for them to experience enough safety and comfort to step into the conversation. Sometimes we take a break in these conversations to go to the restroom, to allow time for reflection, to consult with colleagues or to regroup, take a breath and then reconvene to carry on. At other clinics, there are tight timelines such as three quarters of an hour and you must work efficiently within that time.

Risk assessment is an ongoing part of these conversations as opposed to carried out through a separate assessment tool. Questions that learn about risk and safety and assist people to embrace greater safety are asked throughout the conversation. Safety planning, as needed, often takes place nearing the end of the session, as the plan may look very different by the end than if it was developed early on. Crisis services with a more directive facilitation run parallel to single session practice and can be activated if they would be a better fit and better timed than the therapeutic conversation.

Typically, SST is sought by the participant who wants service to assist with a concern. When it's a therapy sought rather than mandated by authorities, there is no need for exclusionary criteria. Regardless of severity or duration of a problem, we cannot know ahead of time who might find the time useful or who may not. That can only be determined by the participant. I see it as my responsibility to facilitate a process that the participant finds useful. Yet this is not solely on my shoulders as we are in this together, so I can consult with the participant along the way asking what is useful, what should we be doing more or less of, and when enough has been enough. These feedback loops are important and assist us to not lose our way, to maintain focus and be sure we are addressing the agreed upon concern.

This context demands an approach and accompanying skillset that is efficient, focused and that meets people where they are at. A brief narrative approach has proven favourable in navigating the demands of these contexts, not only supporting the skillset required but in spotlighting relational ethics (McNamee, 2009; White, 1997); an ethics of practice[2] that invites continual reflection on the real-life effects of dominant discourse, power relations and the politics of culture influencing the therapeutic encounter.

The emergence of single session therapy as part of a service pathway has found support from three main understandings of the evidence base. First, Hoyt, Rosenbaum, and Talmon (1992) found in review of client contact data the most common number of sessions attended is one! A single session was the most common length of psychotherapy, regardless of therapist orientation, diagnosis, or treatment plan. "We have known for some time the most frequent, or modal, number of therapy sessions is one" (Boyhan 1996; Bloom, 1992, 2001; Talmon, 1990). Given this, perhaps your first thought went to, "Well, maybe they had lousy therapy. They are dropouts!". But that's not the case. What they have come to understand is that many people get what they want or need out of the first session.

Second, the first session in psychotherapy is potentially the most therapeutic and often has the greatest influence on the outcome of therapy, regardless of the total number of sessions used. Review of outcome studies reveals that often the most progress occurs early in psychotherapy, typically first through eighth sessions. This is followed by ever decreasing improvements as psychotherapy continues (Bloom, 2001).

Last, people who use SST are at least as satisfied and show as much improvement (including long-term and ripple effect changes) when compared to people who opted for longer-term therapy (Rosenbaum, Hoyt & Talmon, 1990; Talmon, 1990, 1993; Hoyt, Rosenbaum & Talmon, 1992). People tend to have a very useful experience in single session therapy and a great deal can be accomplished. These findings invite us to seriously consider how do we get direct services to people as soon as possible and how do we make the most out of those first contacts? In part, the answer has been the emergence of mental health walk-in/quick access clinics.

Walk-In Therapy Clinics

The term walk-in[3] therapy and single session therapy are often used interchangeably, as single session practice is most commonly used within walk-in therapy clinics. These clinics have a long history in Canada as first offered in the 1990s at the Eastside Family Centre, in Calgary, Alberta, Canada (Slive, Maclauren, Oakander, Amundson, 1995; Slive, McElheran, & Lawson, 2001). As noted, Karen Young oversaw an urban walk-in clinic at a children's mental health centre which opened in 2000 and our clinic, a rural iteration which I initiated and supervised, opened in 2006. Ours, along with several other clinics began gathering data as to the usefulness of this evolving service pathway. Ontario specifically had become a catalyst for the creation of the walk-in therapy service model. Karen and I worked throughout the years providing training for many new clinics who shared a collective desire to get direct services to children and families as soon as possible, free of wait times and barriers to access such as long assessment tools and screening measures.

In 2014, children's mental health centres throughout Ontario were mandated to provide walk-in therapy clinic services as a part of the transformation of children's mental health. Young (2020) highlights three important developments along the way including a 2012 policy paper (Duvall, Young & Kayes-Burden), a comprehensive evaluation of multiple walk-in therapy clinics (Young & Bhanot-Malhotra, 2014), and an appeal decision accepting single session therapy as psychotherapy by The College of Registered Psychotherapists of Ontario (Young & Jebreen, 2019).

With this momentum, from 2001 through to 2022, three walk-in clinics grew to approximately 90 throughout the province, serving diverse populations (Young, Dick, Herring & Lee, 2008). These clinics are like medical walk-in clinics, with the difference being people come to take part in a single session of psychotherapy. People receive service at their time of need, often free of charge, and free of extensive assessment and wait times. This growth reflected more than just a fad or trend for the time. They emerged because they are useful to people and the feedback and research supports this (Hoyt & Talmon, 2014; Riemer, Booton, Kermani, Horton, Cait, Dittmer & Stalker, 2018).

The process at these clinics involves completion of some pre-session paperwork that intentionally highlights difference and competence upon arrival. That pre-session paperwork is reviewed, and the participant(s) is matched to a therapist. They meet for a complete episode of psychotherapy. A document is co-crafted that serves as the clinical record and is offered to the participant to take with them to extend the influence of the conversation. The intention of this process was to remove barriers to service to get the product to the people and capitalize on the difference often generated within a first session of therapy.

Evolving Brief Narrative Therapy

Narrative therapy is connected under the brief umbrella, as it is an approach widely adapted to time constrained contexts. It is cited as used at walk-in clinics throughout the province of Ontario more often than a Cognitive Behavioural Therapy approach (Duvall, Young & Kays-Burden, 2012). The genre of brief narrative therapy that has emerged has its roots in those live demonstrations previously noted, where Michael White (co-founder of narrative therapy) would meet with people to demonstrate narrative practice during training forums.

Watching those conversations taught us a great deal about how to navigate time constraint. Often, Michael would spend quite a bit of time getting to know people at the outset. He would inquire about the things they liked to do, their work or school, general interests, and the history of those interests. He would share somewhat about himself. To many, this seemed like general conversation but then, as if by magic, pieces of this initial talk would sprout later in the conversation, shaping a useful metaphor or connected to broader skills and values that could be utilized to address the problem they had come about. The most meaningful next steps incorporated these skills and interests people already had experience with. We were learning to meet people through their stories of competence to quickly get on to experiences that could be built upon and brought into preferred storylines.

Throughout the conversation, with permission, Michael would take notes, periodically pausing so he could get the persons' words down just the way they said it. He would repeat phrases back, checking to be sure he had understood it right. Other times he would share back as if re-telling the story they had shared with an emphasis on the material that had emerged outside the problem story. He was teaching us about documenting practices and how these practices can assist re-tellings, meaning making, and the importance of providing reflective space for participants.

His general posture was informed by seemingly insatiable curiosity accompanied by a vast repertoire of questions. Those questions helped to travel to unforeseen places in these conversations; often places which the participant had overlooked. The questions canvassed their experiences and the wisdom they had grown. A description of any preferred event was often followed with an invitation to connect to what it could mean about who the person was becoming, what they stood for or intended for their life. These were not interrogative questions but like invitations pointing to a map asking, look at this for a second, should we go here, what do you think of this, what sense do you make of this place, of what you were able to do, is this exciting to you? These were some of Michael's lessons about collaboration, and the way questions can assist people to research their experience, explore meanings and co-create new or revised understandings.

Nearing the end of the conversations, Michael would ask some interesting questions that invited the participant to speculate and project into the future the possible ripples of what they had discussed. Questions like, "If you were to leave here and have these ideas with you when you needed them, what difference will that make?" and "How will you keep these ideas with you and put them to work when you return home?" were teaching us ways to assist the conversation to live on past the face-to-face, re-contextualized into everyday living.

The lessons drawn from those demonstrations grew narrative practice specific to single session and time constrained settings. As a derivative of narrative therapy, "brief narrative therapy" is not a hurried therapy, but complete and in harmony with the practices and ethics of narrative therapeutic practice.

Brief narrative conversations can involve re-authoring conversations (White & Epston, 1990) assisting people to identify and link the initiatives of their lives into stories-in-the-making more fitting with their preferences for life and identity. Conversations can provide a venue for people to become more acquainted with, and share, their skills for living and wisdom associated with more preferred storylines. Conversations can also quickly pull apart limiting ideas and understandings, assisting people to develop a revised position on a problem or further develop counter practices to the oppression of problems.

All these paths, as White (2006, 2007, 2011) has noted, provide the context in which people can distance from the known and familiar of their lives and move towards their preferred life. When the material of these conversations is brought into proposals for action, the therapy stretches beyond the single contact and can prove quite useful to the people consulting to us.

This approach, like all therapeutic approaches, is informed by understandings about people, problems and change that shape what happens in practice. These understandings shape how we think about our role, understand how people experience and express distress, and conceive of how to facilitate therapeutic conversation. Several key concepts that are favourable to single session encounters inform a brief narrative approach. In the next chapter, I will highlight some of the thinking that shapes my brief narrative practice.

Before that, it is important to note this practice is informed by meta-theory that shapes the approach. In referencing meta-theory, I am referring to a zoomed-out view situating the work within a theoretical backdrop. Post-structuralism, feminism, and post-modernism ideas have significantly influenced narrative therapy. Ideas about meaning generation, language as creational, how identity is socially and relationally shaped, the influence of dominant discourse and attention to power relations all shape how we hear and respond in these conversations. Those responses have effects on people's lives in contributing to how they come to know possibility and know themselves. It is our responsibility to have explored those possible effects and the ethics of our practice. I will not elaborate further on the meta-theory here, as there is a great deal already written that can be explored on this topic (White, 1997, 2001; Russell & Carey, 2004; Tarragona, 2008; Gergen, 2009). I invite you to immerse in the meta-theory to engage in reflection on the possible effects of these theories in shaping your practice and, subsequently, people's lives.

My work is situated within the postmodern, post-structural worlds of meta-theory embracing the subjectivity of meaning and meaning-making process, moving away from imposing grand generalizations and the medicalizing of personal distress. It is this focus on meaning and the meaning generation that serves the time constraint of single session therapy so generously.

Notes

1 By the term "cheerleading" I am referring to the tendency to compliment people or share praise as a means to encourage people to carry on. In SST, this may be haz-ardous as people could perceive compliments as judgement, and encouragement as incongruent with what they see as possible. Given we may not see them again to address any misunderstanding, these are practices we move away from in SST. I do not see it as my role to encourage, compliment, or cheerlead people in therapy. Rather, I may ask questions that assist people to make sense of their experiences on their own.

2 I'll speak more to "relational ethics" and single session therapy in Chapter 2, how-ever I want to note that to me it is a missing conversation in much of the field. With an emphasis on outcomes, the risk is we are not paying attention to how we go about achieving those outcomes; to how we do what we do. Single session therapy, with such time constraint demands special attention to how we do what we do and the pos-sible effects on people's real lives as there may not be an opportunity to address any misunderstanding or mishap.

3 The term "walk-in therapy" is a derivative of medical "walk-in" clinics. However, the term is problematic excluding those with alternate means of mobility. As an alterna-tive, the use of the term "quick access clinic" or "open access" has begun to emerge and is preferable to walk-in. I will use the term walk-in throughout the book for clarity but please know this is not intended to make invisible those with alternate means of mobility.

References

Bloom, B. L. (1992). *Planned short-term psychotherapy*. Boston: Allyn & Bacon.

Bloom, B. L. (2001). Focused single-session psychotherapy: A review of the clinical and research literature. *Brief Treatment and Crisis Intervention, 1*(1),75–86.

Boyhan, P. (1996). Clients' perceptions of single session consultations as an option waiting for family therapy. *Australian and New Zealand Journal of Family Therapy, 17*(2), 85–96.

Cannistrà, F. & Piccirilli, F. (2021). *Single-session therapy: Principles and practice (Psychotherapy in practice)* (K. Croll-Knight, Trans.). Giunti Psychometrics.

Children's Mental Health Ontario. (2020). (rep.). Kids can't wait: 2020 report on wait lists and wait times for child and youth mental health care in Ontario. Retrieved October 16, 2021, from https://cmho.org/wp-content/uploads/CMHO-Report-WaitTimes-2020.pdf.

Dryden, W. (2019). *Single-session therapy (SST): 100 Key Points and techniques.* Routledge.

Duvall, J., Young, K. & Kays-Burden, A. (2012). No more, no less: Brief mental health services for children and youth. Ontario Centre of Excellence for Child and Youth Mental Health, November 2012, retrieved January 2013 www.excellenceforchildandyouth.ca/sites/default/files/policy_brief_mental_health_services_1.pdf

Gergen, K. J. (2009). *An invitation to social construction.* London: Sage.

Hoyt, M. F., Rosenbaum, R. & Talmon, M. (1992). Planned single-session psychotherapy. In: S. H. Budman, M. F, Hoyt, S. Friedman, (Eds.). *The first session in brief therapy.* New York: The Guildford Press.

Hoyt, M. F. & Talmon, M. (2014). *Capturing the moment: Single session therapy and walk-in services.* Bethel, CT: Crown House Publishing Co.

McNamee, S. (2009). Postmodern psychotherapeutic ethics: Relational responsibility in practice. *Human Systems, 20*(2), 55–69

Riemer, M., Booton, J., Kermani, N., Horton, S., Cait, C.-A., Dittmer, L. & Stalker, C. (2018). The walk-in counselling model of service delivery: Who benefits most? *Canadian Journal of Community Mental Health, 37*(2), 29–47. https://doi.org/10.7870/cjcmh-2018-019

Rosenbaum, R., Hoyt, M. F. & Talmon, M. (1990). The challenge of single-session therapies: Creating pivotal moments. In R. A. Wells & V. J. Giannetti (Eds.), *Handbook of brief psychotherapies* (pp. 165–189). Plenum Press.

Russell, S. & Carey, M. (2004). *Narrative therapy: Responding to your questions.* Adelaide, Australia: Dulwich Centre Publications.

Slive, A. & Bobele, M. (2011). *When one hour is all you have: Effective therapy for walk-in clients.* Phoenix, AZ: Zeig, Tucker, & Theisen.

Slive, A., MacLaurin, B., Oakander, M. & Amundson, J. (1995). Walk-in single sessions: A new paradigm in clinical service delivery. *Journal of Systemic Therapies, 14*(1), 3–11. https://doi.org/10.1521/jsyt.1995.14.1.3

Slive, A., McElheran, N. & Lawson, A. (2001). Family therapy in walk-in mental health clinics. In M. MacFarlane (Ed.), *Family therapy and mental health: Innovations in theory and practice* (pp. 261–285). New York: Haworth.

Talmon, M. (1990). *Single-session therapy: Maximizing the effect of the first (and often only) therapeutic encounter.* San Francisco: Jossey–Bass Publishers.

Talmon, M. (1993). *Single-Session Solutions: A guide to practical, effective, and affordable therapy.* Addison-Wesley Pub.

Tarragona, M. (2008). Postmodern/poststructuralist therapies. In J. L. Lebow (Ed.), *Twenty-first century psychotherapies: Contemporary approaches to theory and practice* (pp. 167–205). Wiley.

White, M. (1997). Re-membering. In White, M. (1997) *Narratives of therapists lives.* Adelaide, Australia: Dulwich Centre Publications.

White, M. (2001). Folk psychology and narrative practice. *Dulwich Centre Journal*, (2), 1–37. Reprinted in M. White (2004). *Narrative practice and exotic lives: Resurrecting diversity in everyday life* (pp. 59–118). Adelaide, Australia: Dulwich Centre Publications.

White, M. (2007). *Maps of narrative practice*. New York: W.W. Norton.

White, M. (2011). *Narrative practice: Continuing the conversations*. New York: W.W. Norton.

White, M. & Epston, D. (1990). *Narrative means to therapeutic ends*. New York: W.W. Norton.

White, M. & Morgan, A. (2006). *Narrative therapy with children and their families*. Adelaide, Australia: Dulwich Centre Publications.

Young, K. (2006). *When all the time you have is now: Narrative practice at a walk-in therapy clinic*. Retrieved September 16, 2020, from Narrative Approaches website: https://narrativeapproaches.com/when-all-the-time-you-have-is-now-narrative-practice-at-a-walk-in-therapy-clinic/

Young, K. (2020). Multistory listening: Using narrative practices at walk-in clinics. *Journal of Systemic Therapies*, *39*(3), 34–45.

Young, K. & Bhanot-Malhotra, S. (2014). Getting services right: An Ontario multi-agency evaluation study. Retrieved from Windz Centre Web Site www.windzcentre.com September 5, 2022.

Young, K. & Jebreen, J. (2019). Recognizing single session therapy as psychotherapy. *Journal of Systemic Therapies*, *38*(4), 31–44.

Young, K., Dick, M., Herring, K. & Lee, J. (2008). From waiting lists to walk-in: Stories from a walk-in therapy clinic. *Journal of Systemic Therapies*, *27*(4), 23–39. https://doi.org/10.1521/jsyt.2008.27.4.23

Chapter 2

Key Concepts in Brief Narrative Therapy

A brief narrative therapy is very much in harmony with the tradition of narrative practice (White & Epston, 1990). While the term "brief" has come to be connected to narrative practice as a means to share a therapy that is useful working under time constraint, we do not mean it to imply you simply do narrative practice in less time. In a similar vein to the genre of brief therapy demonstrated at the MRI, brevity in itself has not been the goal but rather brevity comes about as a consequence of how we think about people, problems, change, and therapy and how these premises shape what we do.

We all bring with us implicit assumptions about how we do what we do. Often, they go unnoticed or unarticulated, but regardless, we all have them. They speak to where we locate problems, ideas about how people address their complaints, ideas about who holds knowledge or how knowledge is put to work, and ideas about the process of therapy. In this chapter, I will highlight several of the key concepts of a brief narrative approach within which the remaining chapters are situated. The following is not an exhaustive summary by any means, but a spotlight on key concepts that help to frame the rest of this book within a theoretical backdrop.

Meaning Making

A central concept is that humans are meaning making beings constantly involved in a process of trying to make sense of their world. We filter material that matters from the panorama of life to assist us to navigate our world. Yet, out of all the colours, smells, sounds, and interactions, very little gets noticed and is used to form our concept of the world. What does get noticed and tended to becomes the sense we make of who we are, our relationships and life in general. When people come to therapy, they bring with them the sense they have made of their experiences, those highly filtered understandings they have arrived at through the social process of living a life. When people seek therapy, often those meanings are problematic, limiting and/or not preferred. However, what is exciting about this and particularly useful to single session therapy is that because meaning is

DOI: 10.4324/9781003431688-3

continually constructed in conversation, past meanings can be renegotiated, and new meanings can be co-developed. In a single session, it means when focused on meaning making, there is *always* somewhere to go in these conversations.

My project is to engage people in a meaning-making process through dialogue. As noted, past meanings can be re-negotiated, re-imagined, or new meanings can be co-developed as the conversation unfolds. These conversations are therefore generative of possibility. For instance, a parent who arrived understanding that they were failing their child, not knowing how to handle their tantrums and outbursts, came to a very different conclusion about their parenting following exploration of the many skills that they had taught their child that went unnoticed. Becoming reacquainted with those successes sparked new ideas for how to address tantrums and assisted the parent to come to see themselves as more competent than originally thought.

As another example, a young woman came to the walk-in therapy clinic, distressed by the experience of seeing creatures coming through the walls to torment her. This experience had come on suddenly and following a trip to her doctor, an appointment was scheduled for psychiatry, fearing she needed a diagnosis of schizophrenia. Seeking relief from this, she attended the walk-in where, in conversation, it came forward that an uncle had sexually assaulted her prior to these visual experiences. I asked, "what if you think about this experience of seeing creatures coming through the walls a response to what happened? What kind of response might it be?"

Confused by this different understanding of her experience, she asked, "What do you mean?"

"Well, if we think about what you are seeing as a response of some sort to what you have been through could it be a way of saying I won't be silent about what happened, I will not accept this?"

This question caught her interest as it introduced the "experience of seeing creatures" as a *response*[1] to assault and an act of resistance, expressing that she is not okay with that. She began to put words to this and to see herself as actively responding rather than becoming ill.

A lot is happening in that short conversation engaging in meaning making. I am resisting individualizing the problem as a mental health disorder as it becomes linked to the context of her experience. Beginning to understand her distress as an action on her part, as a means of speaking out, begins to restore a sense of personal agency. The hallucinations abated following this conversation, and she developed plans to address the effects of the assault while she awaited ongoing services.

Story

The concept of story aids us in understanding and navigating the meaning making process with people. Exploring the structure of "story", we are oriented to the events of people's lives that become linked over time according to themes or plots about life, relationships, and self. These stories are meaning making frames that organize lives providing lenses through which people view and interpret events and their lives in general (White & Epston, 1990). In this way, the stories we know and live shape the meanings we ascribe to new events and can be quite limiting or freeing.

Most often, when people come to the walk-in therapy clinic, they share very limiting problem saturated stories. These personal accounts may involve conclusions about life as too difficult, futile, or ideas about themselves, such as with deficits, depressed, or anxiety ridden. They may share broader themes of helplessness, traumatization, or failure. These stories can be limiting in that they influence what events go unnoticed or are pruned from life's panorama of experiences and ascribed meaning. A dominate story can come to speak to who we are, overshadowing, and even eclipsing the material of life that is more preferred, experiences outside the problem definition, or material that's directly counter to the problem. These single-storied accounts come to hide or overshadow that our lives are multi-storied.

Through engaging people's meaning making skills, we invite them to recall and/or reconsider the events of their lives that are more preferred. These exceptions, unique outcomes, initiatives or counter knowledges can be linked to alternate stories or "stories-in-the-making" that are more preferred, hope friendly and provide a foundation for plans of action. I refer to the linking of these preferred events as stories-in-the-making, as they are often not yet well-formed dominate stories but rather emerging storylines/meanings that, when more widely considered and circulated, may come to bring people relief.

Generate Local Knowledge

Working with meaning making through the framework of story means we are drawing extensively from the lived experience, interpretations, and worldview of the participant. As such, we are always engaged in the relational process of knowledge generation in a conversation. It is said that the greatest contribution to change comes from what people bring with them to the process (Duncan, Miller, 2000). The material people arrive with is represented by many concepts such as skills, abilities, strengths, resilience, know-how developed through the years, preferences for how things could be, hopes, wishes, values, beliefs, intentions for life, moral codes, commitments, imagination, and nourishing supportive relationships. White and Epston (1990) distinguish this material from professional knowledge taking up the term "insider knowledge" or "local knowledge" (Geertz, 2000). White speaks to these concepts generally as "… those everyday acts of life that have to do with the making of a 'living', with getting through the day, with the forging of an identity, and with the fabricating of relationships" (White, 2004, p. 98–99).

Yet this material doesn't lie within someone, rather it is generated together in conversation through dialogue, question/response, coming visible as it is voiced out loud or privately to oneself. It is co-constructed, in that it's shared both ways, negotiated, and jointly developed (Sutherland, Fine & Ashbourne, 2012). Generated together, it is informed by the experience that both participant and therapist bring to the process. Facilitating knowledge generation is important to the context of SST, as when ideas are locally informed, they will tend to be something people already know about or how to do, making a better fit for their context and culture.

By mutually generating ideas, people will leave with a sense that they are knowledgeable about their life and circumstances and can affect those circumstances. Local knowledge generation is in contrast to other traditions in which ideas are prescribed, taught, or instructed based on professional universal theories. Further, knowledge generation resists positioning the therapist as the knower; a posture that can inadvertently foster reliance and erase someone's personal agency.

Given this, local knowledges are canvased and discussed in relation to how they assist people. My understanding is that we serve people best when we can draw from them their ideas and competencies to be put to use rather than instructing or teaching. Co-developed knowledge can be brought into take-away documents that assist our conversations to last past the face-to-face contact.

Local knowledge tends to be nuanced and particular. Take the craft of fly fishing. You can gain knowledge from a book about fly fishing or fishing in general however it is very different knowledge than that generated through the lived experience of the activity. From a book, the ideas are more universal, lacking the detail informed by context. It is only from the fisherperson themselves that the contextualized nuances of the activity come available. They can articulate when to fish in which river at a specific time of day, month, or year. They will know how the currents and feeding work in that specific river and thus which lure would be the most productive. They could mentor us in the particular thread used to tie on a specific sized hook depending on location, time, and species they are trying to lure. They could speak to their thrill that keeps them involved in the activity and could share times of discouragement and triumph.

It is that kind of local and specific knowledge that we are seeking in a brief narrative single session encounter. Knowledge is languaged into existence and comes known or more visible through our conversations. I do this by inviting participants to mentor me in their know-how. We are searching in the gaps of the problem storyline for incongruence that may highlight their own wisdom. We are extracting from the problem story itself the lived experiences that are contextually based. We are collecting the skills of everyday living to be brought together as a basis to launch a range of responses. It's a process of co-researching[2] people's lived experience (Epston, 1999, 2001, 2014), inviting them to be the teacher. This knowledge or material is heard within the stories people share. People's lived experiences become the points of entry for inquiry, exploration, and discovery.

Curiosity

Curiosity is at the heart of narrative practice and developing a wide field of curiosity is an important part of time constrained work. It's a curiosity about what matters to people, what they want different and the times they may have experienced that difference even a little, whether in life or imagined. It's a curiosity that undermines notions of certainty, reaching beyond a model driven view that orients to concepts such as symptoms, cognition, regulation, or other internal state metaphors. I am talking about a limitless field of curiosity unbounded by what we think is normal or popular ideas about how people should be living. This curiosity spans the timeline at times reaching far back, loitering in the near now, or stretching into the unwritten future. It's curiosity about people's lived experience that provides the entry points to the material that can be brought into stories-in-the-making.

When it's directed to meaningful preferred events that perhaps were previously out of sight, it invites the participants' own curiosity and interest. Curiosity becomes contagious. They will want to step more fully into the conversation to learn more about what they had done and what it could suggest about what's possible and who they are becoming. Together, we explore possibility and difference. In this way, curiosity is also closely linked to the concept of relationship or therapeutic alliance in SST. When employing a therapy of questions and curiosity, relationship develops through how we respond moment to moment. If I can ask questions that evoke the interest of the participant, relationship grows. Therefore, therapeutic alliance is not a separate project that has to occur before the real work begins. If someone shows up, you have relationship especially given a single session is most often self-selected. The key is not to mess it up. Relationship is continually fostered through how we respond with genuine curiosity.

Together, we can enter into wonder and exploration. We are on the lookout for the moments that lie outside what the problem story would have predicted. As I am curious about these unique outcomes, exceptions, or initiatives, an information gap opens in which the participants' curiosity grows wanting to know more (Storr, 2021). These are gaps that are not too strange or satellite but offshoot from the problem story. For instance, if someone was to say to me, "I've been in so many abusive relationships in my life, it's so hard to know now what a safe relationship is", my curiosity leads to questions such as:

- What were the warning signs you noticed telling you to end many of those relationships?
- What has it made possible to listen to your warning bells and take steps to free your life from those relationships?

- What do your decisions and efforts suggest about the kind of relationships you are seeking?
- How did you come to know to seek those aspects of relationship?

My curiosity directed towards the information gap regarding what is implicitly stated here evokes the others curiosity. Their attention is drawn to that space with my questions as we engage in a mutual dance of meaning making, so to speak.

Questions

Curiosity and questions go hand in hand as our questions reflect the breadth of our curiosity. Questions provide the best way to elicit people's own know-how and invite dialogue favourable to meaning making. With our questions, we are asking people to mentor us in what they bring to the process that can inform a preferred story-in-the-making. As such, our questions are intentional, seeking to elicit and learn more about people's experience of the problem, competencies, preferred developments, intentions, and hopes for the future. Our questions are not meant for information gathering to assess their fit to some cultural norm for how to live.

In asking questions, we are actively proposing domains to explore, such as events from the past, present as we know it, and/or within a speculated future. Clandinin and Connelly (2000) propose the metaphor of a three-dimensional inquiry space to represent narrative inquiry. The domain of temporality is accompanied by the dimension of the personal/social and the dimension of place. I consider the dimension of place as inclusive of context, including culture and spirituality. We can ask questions pointing in many different yet connected ways within these dimensions, inward/outward experiences, backward/forward through time, and located in place, relationship, and culture. We can "explore the possibilities, differences, and contradictions of events that make up 'the passage of time'" (Walther & Carey, 2009, p. 6).

I've always appreciated the idea of asking about difference as likened to tapping someone on the shoulder to say, "Hey, look over here for a minute." Our questions direct attention towards certain experiences and away from other experiences. As our questions seek to learn about unique outcomes and exceptions, people are invited to reflect on and research their experiences. In these moments of recall, revisiting more preferred circumstances, people are generating experience and re-experiencing the preferred events. Answering a question is thus experiential. Questions are used to generate experience.

In raising questions, we are offering novel ways to look at problems and talk about experiences. For instance, as we ask questions that externalize a problem, we are proposing ways to talk differently about experiences, separating from stock plot discussions. Questions assist people to reflect on their lives from different vantage points, which may invite the revision of past meanings.

A Three-Dimensional Inquiry Space

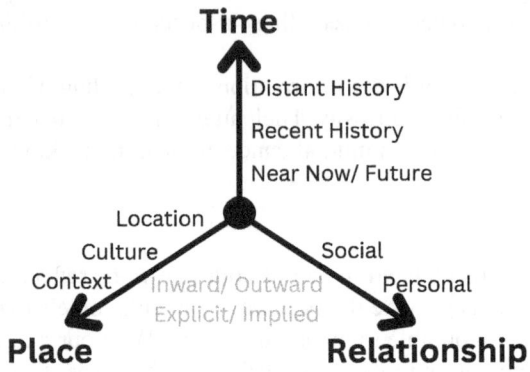

Figure 2.1 A Three-dimensional Inquiry Space adapted from Clandinin and Connelly (2000) illustrating the multiple dimensions within which a question can be situated.

Questions are not neutral in their influence, either. Some questions are better than others within single session therapy. They are not free of meta-message; that unsaid yet communicated messaging. For instance, explore the meta-message in the question: How have you resisted those thoughts about killing yourself? This question presupposes the person has resisted the thoughts, orients them towards that resistance and implies that they exercised some agency in that action. As noted, the question offers domains for exploration and meanings to be co-developed.

Yet, staying curious and developing the "habit of asking questions" can be difficult as the complexity and vexing aspects of problems can have therapists revert to statements, instruction, critique and comment, closing down dialogue. These can be troublesome practices in the context of a single session therapy as they risk centring the therapist's agenda and positioning the therapist as the knower.

Throughout this book, we will explore many questions fitting brief narrative single session therapy that can inform the habit of asking. White (2007) has proposed several maps that serve to collect and organize questions that orient towards specific domains for inquiry. Maps, as an orienting metaphor, group questions that take us places in these conversations while not specifying a fixed or predetermined outcome. They assist us in finding our way through the complexity of content.

Language as Creational

Words-like universes travelling by...

(Tom Andersen, 2012, p.31)

Tom Andersen's poetic words in the above quote speak to a significant shift in the field through the 1990s that also represents an important tenet of brief narrative single session work. It involves the recognition that the language we use is not an exact representation of what it is referring to. Rather, any use of language, spoken or unspoken communication, involves a relational and creational process shaping meaning. We may ascribe any spoken word multiple meanings depending on one's experience, the context within which it's spoken, and how it is received. For instance, if I were to invite you to think of the colour blue, your colour blue will differ from my colour blue. As Andersen implies, words are likened to universes of meanings traveling by and available for exploration. With story as the frame for meaning and dependent on language, we are ascribing meaning to our experience and constituting our lives and relationships through language (White & Epston, 1990).

In a single session therapy and therapy in general then, the language we use is therefore not neutral but life shaping. Words do things to people. They can hold us in meaning that is common and familiar or take us down different paths to revised or new landscapes of meaning and possibility. We use language to exercise people's meaning making skills, to generate knowledge and broaden the field of possibility, invoke presupposition, invite multiple perspectives, and language into existence preferred meanings.

Languaging

I have found it useful to think about our conversations as "languaging" (Manturana, 1978). Switching from a noun to a verb, language is a generative action of co-creation of meaning. In dialogue, we listen to ourselves speak and simultaneously watch for how we are being received to adjust how we are speaking in the moment. In this exchange, we are actively co-shaping meanings with participants. For me, this represents more clearly the social process and creational aspect of language in therapy and foregrounds our part of the process. We then have to take responsibility for the possible effects of our words and words in general in shaping knowledge and one's experience, especially when we may only meet with someone once. As we understand the "productive potential" (Tilsen, 2018) of language, consider "what are we languaging into existence" so to speak, through our interaction? Said another way, what storying am I taking part in?

It's an invitation to root out and resist replicating the politics of culture through language that invites patriarchy, normalizing judgement, pathology or colonizes into model speak rather than facilitates preferred story development. In the micro-practices, we are resisting naming problems for people and instead draw forward their own words and descriptions.

Our use of language has intention as we use words to co-create worlds. For instance, shifting adjectives to nouns as in an externalizing conversation (see Chapter 10) where problems are discussed as separate from people, co-creates a world where the problem becomes an antagonist and participant the protagonist. Pre-suppositional language brings into focus a place where difference is possible. Agency can be found through implication, asking "how did you do that"? Tending to language in this way, with a spirit of exchange, wonder, and imagination, is generative of possibility. Again, it also invites us to monitor the possible effects of the words we use in contributing to meaning making, holding us to account for how we do what we do.

Identity Projects

People are constantly making sense of themselves through their relationships and drawing conclusions about "who they are". The therapeutic space is not exempt from this. Michael White, co-founder of narrative therapy, used to say often that we are always involved in identity projects. He was speaking of how identity is socially and relationally shaped in these conversations. For me, this is an important theoretical move away from ideas about a fixed identity, personality, or pre-determined characteristics that a modernistic meta-theory would propose.

To embrace this understanding means we bear great responsibility for how people come to know themselves through a single session conversation. Understanding identity as fluid or as always becoming, the notion of migration of identity (White, 1995) is useful. This refers to how through these conversations people are moving from one way of knowing themselves towards a more preferred way. Past conclusions or ascribed identities become left behind as people consider and embrace more preferred ideas about who they are.

Within these conversations, I want to ask questions that assist people to experience themselves as successful, competent, and able to direct their lives. Exploring this landscape of identity (White, 2007) involves asking questions that invite people to make meaning and interpretations of the preferred events of their lives. What might the preferred developments say about who they are becoming? What might their actions speak to about what's important to them? What is it like to know that so much about them lives outside the problem description?

Understanding the unfolding identity project in a single session means we are not bound by any particular description. Facilitating conversations in which people can come to know themselves in more preferred ways is the enactment of an ethic. It's a commitment to resisting inducting people into psychotherapy models and locating problems inside of people representing or defining who they are. Constellations of meanings are available to explore, opening far-reaching possibilities for proceeding in life after the face-to-face contact.

Problems as Outside of People

The understanding that problems exist outside of people is a hallmark of narrative practice and exceptionally suited for single session conversations.

Locating problems as outside of people sees people as in relationship with problems, setting the stage for conversations that have people experience themselves as active agents with choice in shaping their lives. As problems are talked about as outside of people and understood as products of culture and history, we are alerted to how they are socially constructed and created over time. This is facilitated through the practice of "externalizing conversations" (White & Espton, 1990). Externalizing conversations are useful in single session therapy as they quickly introduce people to novel ways to consider their experience and provide a different vantage point from which to view their circumstances. We can invite people to talk about problems differently, as entities that can be held up, looked at, and investigated for how they mess with people, relationships, and lives.

Just as important, externalizing conversations are a type of identity conversation. In this practice, we are separating from internalized understandings of problems as an illness, aberration of the brain or some dysfunction in coping. Those conceptions are linked to notions of the self as fixed or static. Externalizing serves as a counter to totalizing identities ascribed through negative labeling and the medicalization of distress. As the problem is discussed as separate from the person's identity, context or what people have been through is brought back into the conversation. A range of ways to respond come available that previously remained unimaginable, including ideas for addressing oppressive contexts. These possibilities for proceeding can inform plans and next steps to put into action the minute people leave.

Therapist Position/Being in the Conversation

Participating in these conversations is special, as people are very generous in sharing with us about their lives when they have only just met us. However, there are unavoidable power relations in the therapeutic context that are at risk of being amplified within single session therapy. Often, the practitioner is viewed as the fixer or helper and is presumed to hold the knowledge to be taught to others. As a means to address this, I have moved away from characterizing the relationship as client/professional. Freire (2011) teaches us that "…dialogue cannot exist without humility" (p.90). At the point of encounter there are not "perfect sages", there are "…only people attempting together, to learn more than they now know" (p. 90).

I am not engaging in a process to "help" the other person. In the helping tradition, I may collude with oppressing a person's experience, knowledge generation, and personal agency. For instance, consider the meta-message of adopting a "helping" posture. How can I help you? I just want to be as helpful as possible. The risk is that they understand this as implying they need our help, which is difficult to know given we are meeting for the first time. It possibly implies I have what they need and structures our time as one of teaching, instructing, or fixing. Lastly, it risks positioning me as the one doing the work, backgrounding the other's personal agency. This is even more sensitive in working with youth and people whose voice has been marginalized through others' actions or organizational structures and policies. Remember, language does things.

To do my best to guard against these risks, I have taken the idea of striving to be *useful* to people. Positioning to be useful invites structuring our time together as a place where I bring something to the process that the participant can choose to use or not. It speaks to my view of the participant as knowing themselves best and able to make decisions for their life. De-centering myself further I seek to position "the conversation" as most useful. I may say, my hope is that this conversation is useful in some way. What would be most useful to talk about? In this way, what I bring to the conversation is know-how in facilitating a process, not preconceived notions about what the person needs to do differently or ideas about how they should be thinking or living their life.

Foregrounding Relational Ethics

How we show up in these conversations is a matter of ethics. I am not referring to the notion of "rule-based ethics" (White, 2011) having to do with adhering to standards of practice or "content ethics" (Swim, George & Wulff, 2001) related to general conduct guides or requirements to adherence to a technique. While those notions of ethics can be important, to me, there is a missing conversation. For our purposes we see "… ethics as activities that connect oneself with Others" (Andersen, 2001, p. 11). They are about "…how power operates and how it affects people" (Tilsen, 2018, p. 37). In SST there is tremendous responsibility to give attention to how we are with Others as we may not have the opportunity to see someone again to repair a mishap or misunderstanding.

We embrace the notion of *relational ethics* (McNamee, 2009; White, 2011) in brief narrative therapy. Under the umbrella of collaborative ethics (White, 2011), relational ethics direct our attention to the possible *effects of what we do* on shaping people's real lives, how they come to know themselves, and what is possible, rather than our ability to execute a technique or achieve a specific outcome. They focus attention to the process of being in relationship with the Other. Attention to relational ethics means we are continually monitoring how we do what we do in SST and the possible effects on people's lives. It's through our relational ethics that we strive to facilitate a socially just therapy, recognizing as Paré (2014)[3] does, the "consequential nature of talk" especially as it relates to identity construction. He proposes pro-justice practices such as keeping context visible, attending to responses, inviting evaluation of diagnoses, and separating person and problem.

With relational ethics in the foreground, SST processes may have been hazardous if we have inadvertently engaged in:

- Colonizing practices: pathologizing, categorizing, inducting people into models of therapy, reinforcing colonial ideologies and dominant Western cultural ideals.
- Replicated the politics of culture: participated in dominant culture stories that serve to oppress such as heterosexual dominance, gender binaries, patriarchy, individualism.
- Centred the therapists' agenda: losing sight of what the participant wants and pursuing the therapists' ideas about what they need.
- Participated in normalizing judgment: assisting people to conform to normative social demands and expectations.
- Privileged outsider knowledge: become instructional to the point of backgrounding people's own knowledge.
- Obscured a person's sense of personal agency: talking in a way that makes it hard for people to know they can direct and shape their lives.

Recognizing that there is no perfect therapy, foregrounding relational ethics assists to inoculate, as best we can, against these circumstances and invites us to be accountable for how we participate in these conversations. Our relational responsibility is elevated alongside or beyond our individual responsibility as outlined by outside authorities.

Vikki Reynolds,[4] an activist/therapist residing in British Columbia, Canada, calls for us to centre ethics at the heart of practice (Reynolds, 2010, 2012). This means first and foremost being responsible for addressing power, doing solidarity, critically engaging with language, and structuring safety in practice (Reynolds, 2012). Again, to me, this has been the missing conversation in the field, that is, attention to the possible effects of talk. Through this lens, how we do what we do, the process, is equally as important as outcomes. Chapter 18 will introduce a process/outcome tool that assists to keep practice ethics visible in single session therapy.

Therapy as a Definitional Ceremony

With attention to relational ethics, and in moving away from the traditional client/professional dichotomy, a re-conceptualization of our time together in general is useful. With great attention to meaning making, generation of local knowledge, and identity, the therapeutic context of single session therapy has moved away from the traditional psychological process of treatment, towards ceremony. This ceremony, known as a definitional ceremony, marks a transition to a revised status or role. "We work to make the therapy conversation a ritual space in which the performance of meaning can occur" (Freedman & Coombs, 2002, p.32).

Ceremony involves coming together in a social arena to hear, witness, and build upon what people are already doing and knowing. As such, people have an opportunity to make visible and have witnessed that which has been made invisible, been overshadowed, or not brought into story lines. People are involved in an experience of co-authoring alternative stories of life.

Definitional ceremony is also concerned with identity, providing a venue for people to come to know themselves differently. Within this arena people can become known on their own terms in ways that fit with their preferences.

As a ceremony of sort, brief narrative SST is a whole therapy with a beginning, middle, and ending reflecting change as movement. People depart from old ways of doing and thinking, moving towards revised action, and meaning. This re-conceptualization of the therapeutic encounter has important implications for SST. I will elaborate on this in Chapter 3.

Summary

I have begun to lay the foundation of thinking favourable to generative and useful single session encounters influenced through a brief narrative practice lens. Again, this is not an exhaustive outline and further thinking will be highlighted within related chapters. These ideas are presented to provide a starting framework for the remainder of the material shared. This mind-set and related practices are linked to important relational practice ethics. We cannot separate our thinking and practice from ongoing reflection on the possible effects on people's real lives and understanding of identity.

Adopting these assumptions as a guide, in summary, brief narrative intention informs a quick access/walk-in clinic organizational culture that:

- Recognizes the importance of how meaning is socially and relationally shaped and affects how people respond to the world.
- Employs practices that support the development of personal agency (a person's sense that they can do something about the problem) and increased options for proceeding (a person's sense of knowing what to do about the problem).
- Privileges insider knowledge (know-how) in that what the participants bring with them to the process is further languaged into existence and utilized in addressing the concern or in moving life towards their preferred view.
- Collaborates in developing plans and next steps. These are co-developed and co-shaped building primarily from the participants' own knowledge and experiences.
- Serves to provide ways in which the conversation can be sustained following the visit such as through developing plans and next steps that are culturally and contextually relevant and archived in "take away documents" for people to review afterwards.

The subsequent chapters will share in more detail a brief narrative approach to time constrained conversations, even in very complex circumstances.

Notes

1 The work of Linda Coates, Allan Wade, and Cathy Richardson informs what they refer to as response-based practice. This work is in harmony with our brief narrative practice and has important implications for therapeutic practice in general. See (Wade, 1997; Todd & Wade, 2004; Coates & Wade, 2015). A few publications are available on their website www.responsebasedpractice.com

2 David Epston, (2014) notes how anthropological enquiry has influenced narrative therapy in which the "local knowledge" later called "insider knowledge" of the person consulting is canvassed. Therapeutic inquiry is likened to co-research with participants, the co-production of knowledge by participant and therapist.

3 David Paré is a wonderful writer, academic, and skilled supervisor in Canada. Many of his writings are available at the Glebe Institute website www.glebeinstitute.com. You may find many of his contributions relevant to single session therapy and practice ethics.

4 I believe, Vikki Reynolds is one of the most important voices in the field at this time. Many of her publications are available at her website www.vikkireynolds.ca and I encourage you to acquaint with her extensive work. Although not written specifically for single session therapy, she brings to the conversation important considerations for the future of practice.

References

Andersen, T. (2001). Ethics before ontology: A few words. *Journal of Systemic Therapies*, *20*(4), 11–13. https://doi.org/10.1521/jsyt.20.4.11.23089

Andersen, T. (2012). Word–universes traveling by. In T. Malinen, S. J. Cooper, & F. N. Thomas (Eds.), *Masters of narrative and collaborative therapies: The voices of Andersen, Anderson, and White* (pp. 17–60). Routledge.

Clandinin, D. J. & Connelly, F. M. (2000). *Narrative inquiry: Experience and story in qualitative research*. Jossey-Bass Publishers.

Coates, L. & Wade, A. (2015). We're in the 21st century after all: Analysis of social responses in individual support and institutional reform. In M. Hyden, D. Gadd, & A. Wade (Eds.), *Response-based approaches to the study of interpersonal violence*. London: Palgrave MacMillan.

Duncan, B. & Miller, S. (2000). *The heroic client: Doing client-directed, outcome informed therapy*. San Francisco: Jossey-Bass.

Epston, D. (1999). *Co-research: The making of an alternative knowledge*. The Dulwich Centre. Retrieved July 3, 2022, from https://dulwichcentre.com.au/articles-about-narrative-therapy/co-research-david-epston/

Epston, D. (2001). Anthropology, archives, co-research and narrative therapy. In D. Denborough (Ed.), *Family therapy: Exploring the field's past, present and possible futures* (pp. 161–166). Dulwich Centre Publications.

Epston, D. (2014). Ethnography, co-research and insider knowledges. *Australian and New Zealand Journal of Family Therapy*, *35*(1), 105–109. https://doi.org/10.1002/anzf.1048

Freedman, J. & Combs, G. (2002). *Narrative therapy with couples... and a whole lot more! A collection of papers, essays and exercises*. Adelaide, Australia: Dulwich Centre Publications.

Freire, P. (2011). *Pedagogy of the oppressed: 30th anniversary edition*. New York: Continuum International Publishing Group.

Geertz, C. (2000). *Local knowledge*. New York: Basic Books.

Manturana, H. R. (1978). Biology of language: The epistemology of reality. In G. A. Miller, E. Lenneberg, & E. H. Lenneberg (Eds.), *Psychology and biology of language and thought: Essays in honor of Eric Lenneberg* (pp. 27–63). Academic Press. www.enolagaia.com/M78BoL.html

McNamee, S. (2009). Postmodern psychotherapeutic ethics: Relational responsibility in practice. *Human Systems, 20*(2), 55–69.

Paré, D. A. (2014). Social justice and the word: Keeping diversity alive in therapeutic conversations. *Canadian Journal of Counselling and Psychotherapy 48*(3), 206–217.

Reynolds, V. (2010). Doing justice as a path to sustainability in community work. Retrieved online July 10, 2012, from www.vikkireynolds.ca

Reynolds, V. (2012). An ethical stance for justice-doing in community work and therapy. *Journal of Systemic Therapies, 31*(4), 18–33. https://doi.org/10.1521/jsyt.2012.31.4.18

Storr, W. (2021). *The science of storytelling: Why stories make us human and how to tell them better*. Abrams Press.

Sutherland, O., Fine, M., & Ashbourne, L. (2012). Core competencies in social constructionist supervision? *Journal of Marital and Family Therapy, 39*(3), 373–387. https://doi.org/10.1111/j.1752-0606.2012.00318.x

Swim, S., St. George, S. A., & Wulff, D. P. (2001). Process ethics: A collaborative partnership. *Journal of Systemic Therapies, 20*(4), 14–24. https://doi.org/10.1521/jsyt.20.4.14.23087

Tilsen, J. B. (2018). *Narrative approaches to youth work: Conversational skills for a critical practice*. Routledge.

Todd, N. & Wade, A. (2004). 'Coming to terms with violence and resistance: From a language of effects to a language of responses', in T. Strong & D. Pare (eds), *Furthering talk: Advances in the discursive therapies*. New York: Kluwer Academic Plenum.

Wade, A. (1997). Small acts of living: Everyday resistance to violence and other forms of oppression. *Contemporary Family Therapy, 19*(1), 23–39.

Walther, S. & Carey, M. (2009). Narrative therapy, difference and possibility: Inviting new becomings. *Context*, Oct.

White, M. (1995). *Re-authoring lives: Interviews & essays*. Adelaide, Australia: Dulwich Centre Publications.

White, M. (2004). Working with people who are suffering the consequences of multiple trauma: A narrative perspective. *International Journal of Narrative Therapy and Community Work*, (1), 45–76. Reprinted in D. Denborough, (Ed.) (2006).

Trauma: Narrative responses to traumatic experience (pp. 25–85). Adelaide, Australia: Dulwich Centre Publications.

White, M. (2007). *Maps of narrative practice*. New York: W.W. Norton.

White, M. (2011). *Narrative practice: Continuing the conversations*. W.W. Norton, New York.

White, M. & Epston, D. (1990). *Narrative means to therapeutic ends*. New York: W.W. Norton.

Chapter 3

Re-Visioning the Therapeutic Context

Portrayals of therapy through media, such as television or movies, often shape people's perceptions and expectations about therapy. Those portrayals, reflective of popular culture, promote characterizations of the process that centre the therapist as the knower, possessing some greater understanding of how to fix a person's life to bring it more in line with what's within "normal" expectations. The discourses and politics of popular Western culture have shaped these portrayals and expectations and are reflected in many well-established therapies.

For instance, meta-discourse such as individualism invites people into seeking personal gain, striving to progress, reflected as "goal talk" in therapy. It requires the location of problems within the individual and emphasizes personal accountability, reparation, and repair (Beaudoin, 2004). Capitalism invites participation in comparison, evaluation, and competition. Individuals are measured and performance evaluated through the use of psychological tools. Patriarchy dictates ideas about how people should preform gender according to long held ideas about masculinity and femininity and supports notions of hierarchy in the therapeutic relationship. The therapist is positioning as the knower, legitimizing instruction about the need to be more mindful, adjust cognitions, or grow self-compassion, depending on the selected theory.

To be clear, I am not trying to enter into a good/bad dichotomy regarding these practices. In different therapeutic contexts in which ongoing review can take place, they may be useful to some people. What I am trying to make visible is that in SST, where you may not see the person again to address any misunderstanding or mishaps, the therapy room as a place to teach, repair, or instruct can become problematic. When unnamed and unexamined for the effects these often taken for granted ways of practice may have on shaping people's lives and how they come to think about themselves, the SST risks becoming illusionary help and narrow in generating possibility.

Yet, much of the SST literature has noted how many diverse therapy models are used within a broader competency-based methodology. I contend that therapists draw from their preferred approach, various metaphors, activities, or ideas to introduce novel conversation. However, within a just practice, this is done

DOI: 10.4324/9781003431688-4

with a tentative voice presenting material as one idea amongst many and seeking feedback from participants about the fit of the content for them. Without a tentative voice, there is a risk of inadvertently colonizing people into models which may not fit contextually or culturally.

It's through the examination of the therapeutic context and the ways in which culture is reproduced that White (2011) invites a re-visioning of that context "that lead[s] to the dismantling of some of the accepted structures and practices of therapy, and that point to the creation of contexts that open new possibilities for dissent" (p. 45). Gergen, a skilled social constructionist, too, calls into question traditions of psychotherapy (Sermijn & Gergen, 2017, p. 60).

> The traditional practices of asking questions, and careful empathic listening, are severely limited. We are *multi-beings* and if you bring only a single way of being into therapy–the result of training in a specific school of therapy–you are reducing your capacity for effective therapeutic relations.

Answering, in part, Whites' invitation, SST and quick access therapy clinics, while still vulnerable to reproducing well circulated cultural practices have set the stage for a transformation in how we conceive of our work, what we do in practice, and have pushed what we understand as possible in time constraint. At my clinic we often move out of the "session room" to converse as we walk a trail along a pond surrounded by nature. My staff can be seen engaged in activity with visitors. Sometimes, they might be using balance boards or immersed in play, testing how long a child can tolerate distress in a room on their own to outlast fears. Other clinics have tea at the kitchen table, hosting conversations in a safe and private relaxed setting. Dedicated space in nature can provide a backdrop for these talks. The burden of assessment and paperwork is lean, getting it out of the way of change conversations.

In this work, we are separating from a past that emphasized assessment, diagnosis, instruction, and prescription, while stepping more fully into a future involving generative, collaborative, co-created conversation. It is a one conversation at a time approach in which we are striving to get the most out of the time together (Slive & Bobele, 2011). In these time-constrained conversations we resist replicating the politics of dominant culture and strive for a more just therapy.

Therapy as a Definitional Ceremony

In moving away from the traditions of psychotherapy, I understand my time spent with individuals and families as akin to a ceremony, specifically a definitional ceremony. A definitional ceremony is a specific kind of ceremony that is used to establish, mark, or define something. Examples in life include the swearing in of police officers or an official, marriage ceremonies, graduations, or coming of age ceremonies. This idea is evoked by Whites' concept of therapy and community work as likened to "definitional ceremonies" which he drew from anthropologist, Barbara Myerhoff (1982) and her ethnographic accounts of working with the Jewish Elders in Los Angeles. Myerhoff, in Turner and Bruner (1986), explains how definitional ceremonies deal with the problems of invisibility and marginality, assisting people to be seen on and in one's own terms through the performance of collective enactments of common values, hopes and preferences. Said another way, they assist to shore up and circulate preferred identities to an audience.

SST as a definitional ceremony is a specific event convened to redefine and *mark* who one is becoming and what might be possible. It marks the beginning of a revised phase of life. Whereas people often arrive at the walk-in experiencing the dominate problem story as eclipsing their competence, defining a negative identity, making invisible their skills, abilities, hopes and values and overlooking how they have carried on despite difficult circumstances, therapy as definitional ceremony makes visible what has been made invisible. It can inform new proposals for action and invoke revised accounts of identity that fit more closely with how people would like to be seen.

The process of these definitional ceremonies involves coming together, sharing stories, performance of possibilities, witnessing, responding in specific ways, and inviting re-tellings and performance to an extended audience. I play an important part in that process not only as the host, senior partner, and facilitator, but also as witness to people's distress, hopes, and successes.

My role as witness to these stories is important recognizing meaning and identity are relationally shaped. Let me add though that witnessing differs from being an audience. Shotter (2009) reminds us that one's "… appearance in the human world as another person of worth depends on your responsiveness to [their] expressions" (p. 1).

As a witness to people's stories, I have a responsibility to respond. This book will explore many ways to respond to people's expressions that assist them to know their worth and the expanded possibilities for their lives. I respond in ways that grow the more preferred storylines of people's lives. At times, I'm required to respond in ways outside of our conversation where I have the responsibility to address social injustice, oppression, and/or danger.

Re-conceptualizing the therapeutic encounter as a definitional ceremony opens new possibilities for what can be achieved in these conversations. Whereas psychological traditions built on assumptions of deficit and repair are concerned with information gathering, assessment, and problem solving, therapy as definitional ceremony becomes intimately linked to an identity project, change as movement, and a focus on the performance of difference. As a forum for the performance of difference, the encounter can even move beyond question and answer, into co-shaping, co-development, co-crafting what might be and its rehearsal.

With this conceptualization I am trying to stress the transformational opportunity that emerges as we join with people in a joint project seeking what might be possible rather than trying to help or fix. The future of single session therapy will be far from the formulaic execution of therapeutic models. I believe it will stand on creativity, metaphor, and the conversational performance of collective activity that has people touch, even for a moment, a preferred life. For now, to add some structure to this project we turn to the rites of passage metaphor.

Therapy as a Rite of Passage

Commonly associated with ceremonies in life, the Rites of Passage metaphor drawn from anthropological literature and the work of French anthropologist Arnold van Gennep (1909, 1960) is a model or metaphor for understanding the process of social and cultural change. It foregrounds concepts of movement, transition, and journey within the notion of life as a series of "rites of passage". The rites of passage as quoted by Turner (1969) are "rites which accompany every change of place, state, social position and age" (p.94). They involve ritual processes of transitions between life stages or statuses. Van Gennep has shown that all rites, whether it be marriage, adoption, funerals, initiations, baptisms, or friendship rites, to name a few, involve movement across three thresholds. Said another way, they involve movement through three phases; the separation phase, transition or liminal phase, and a reincorporation phase.

When applied as a guiding framework for single session therapy, the Rites of Passage opens exciting new conversations for working with the experience of distress, trauma, crisis, substance misuse and transitions in life. Several narrative and competency-based practitioners have applied the rites of passage metaphor to therapeutic contexts. I was first introduced to it through the work of Michael Durrant (1993) who contextualizes live-in treatment as a rite of passage building upon youth's competencies. White and Epston (1990) relate the experience of crisis to the metaphor, which I will explore further in a later chapter. White (1995) takes up the metaphor for the journey of separation from intimate partner violence in relationships. He later evokes it again as a metaphor when being consulted to by people who want to break from addiction and/or excessive consumption of substances (White, 2000). Duvall and Béres (2011) evoke the metaphor to highlight an examination of the process of therapy as opposed to an outcome only focus.

Let's take a brief look at the three phases and then I will detail more specifically in Chapters 5 through 7 how they inform a structure for brief narrative SST.

Phase 1: Separation

The separation phase is the beginning stage of the process of social and cultural change. It involves preparation and a distinct untethering from the way things are in a social structure and/or from ideas of identity. It can be unsettling as the person leaves behind their familiar ways of life, community, and previous identity.

When someone attends a single session, that action is an act of separation. Attendance marks the beginning of a transition from the old ways of doing and viewing. We can talk about this action as "starting out on a new path", "taking a step", "embarking on a new life journey", or "starting a project". These movement metaphors provide a sense of possibility and set the stage for change as movement. This idea will have implications for how we hear and understand the problem story. Any complaint can be seen as an action, beginning separation and implying movement towards a more preferred life.

Phase 2: Liminal

The second stage is the transition or liminal, where people take part in the ritual and experience themselves in new ways. In this space, they are in a state of in-between, neither fully belonging to the past nor fully belonging to the future. They are leaving behind who they were and yet are not who they will become. Metaphorically, imagine the space between silence and speech or the ideas between simplicity and complexity. Picture the space between when a trapeze artist lets go of one trapeze and before they catch the receiving trapeze.

This is a place of discomfort and at times confusion and disorganization (White & Epston, 1990). Within the liminal, how people know themselves becomes increasingly ambiguous. It's within this space that people come to learn things about themselves and the world. They apprentice. This may involve struggle, adjustment, and growth within an atmosphere of exploration and discovery.

In practice, our focus is on "distancing practices"; the journey of incrementally distancing from problem saturated descriptions towards possibility and difference. In facilitating this process, we offer questions and maps of questions to orient and assist people to explore events and the meaning of those events. We may expand entry points to possibility, enter re-authoring conversations, enter externalizing conversations, co-develop counter-stories, or draw upon other domains of inquiry to facilitate this process.

Phase 3: Reincorporation

The last stage "reincorporation" involves arrival with a new or revised identity and/or reconnection to community. With it comes new responsibilities and privileges. There is a commitment to a new path, a determination to carry on and the revised status is declared to an audience. It is often marked by celebration and stepping back into community.

For our purposes in therapeutic practice, this phase directs us to mark arrival at a new or revised understanding of events and/or view of self. With a focus on reincorporation, we facilitate a process that assists people to re-contextualize our conversation back into their everyday living into doable actions. In a sense, the hard work is just beginning and this phase sets the stage for experimentation and practice in the real world after the session. Further, it's a time to identify fitting relationships or audience to the change who can play their part in supporting and shouldering up as needed. In this phase we use the practices of session re-telling, co-developing next steps and the use of take-away documentation to assist the conversation to find audience, endure and mark the moment.

Many have proposed "phases" for representing the therapeutic encounter to orient therapists in conversations. Regarding brief and single session therapy, I'm drawn to Hoyts' 5-phase interpretation (Hoyt, M. 2000) and Duvall and Béres therapy as a three-act play (Duvall in Brown & Augusta-Scott, 2007; Duvall & Béres, 2011) as well as Ray and Keeneys' (1993) three acts relating a session to a theatrical play. My understanding is that Hoyt, Duvall and Béres, and Ray and Keeney each share useful guides for navigating therapy encounters.

I've crafted the following visual conceptualization, a chorography of sort, stepping more fully into the rites of passage analogy. Like the others, it is overly simplified and intended to direct attention to process and specific micro-skills at different times in the conversation. It serves to arrange the parts, offering a guide to the process. This is useful as sometimes the content of a single session can be moving or evocative, making it hard to know how to proceed, having us lose our way in the conversation. A choreography is useful in directing attention to the micro skills and processes to assist the therapist to not get lost or disoriented within the content of what is expressed. It helps us understand where we are in the conversation.

Figure 3.1 highlights the three main phases I have embraced, including the separation, liminal, and arrival phases. This visual reads from the bottom to the top. Simplifying the application, we focus on beginnings, middles, and endings of our brief narrative single session encounter. As people arrive mired in the problem story, they share a very narrow description of their distress represented by the small end of the triangle. I'm disordered, deficited, unable, or a failure are the kinds of narrow representations we may hear in this early part of the process. As time unfolds, in answering our questions, meanings expand into stories-in-the-making that open new proposals for action, forming a horizon of possibilities represented by the larger end of the triangle.

Understanding change as movement, I view the person/family as incrementally distancing from the known and familiar of their life and moving towards the horizon of possibility where new ways of proceeding in life come available and inform action plans. Each phase focuses on specific micro skills that assist

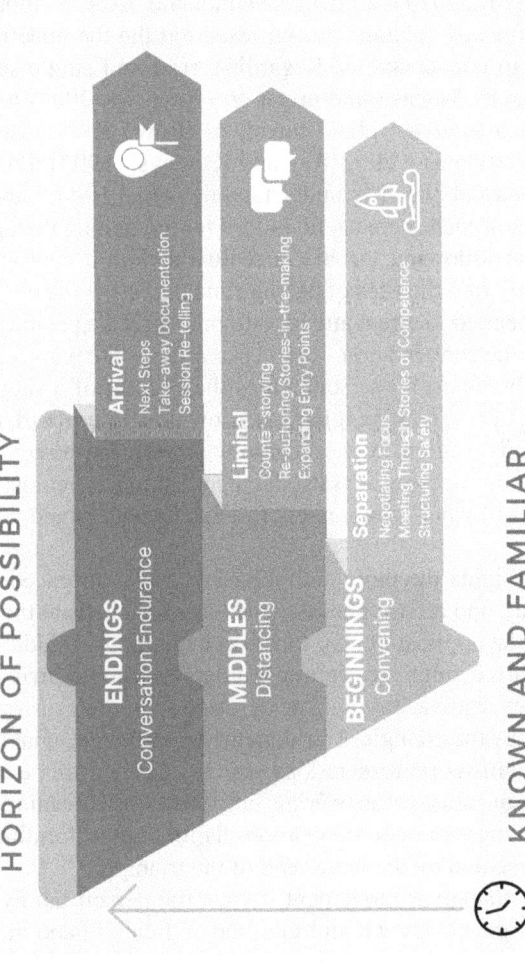

Figure 3.1 The Brief Narrative SST Conversation Map shows the structure of a brief narrative single session conversation. This map reads from the bottom to the top.

Adapted from Van Gennep, 1960; Ray and Keeney, 1993; Hoyt, M. 2000; Duvall & Béres, 2011

in this process. Phase one focuses on what David Epston has referred to as the "acts of convening" that ensure a safe enough context and begin the process with focus. Phase two focuses attention on distancing practices; conversations that assist people in negotiating meanings and discuss preferred events in meaningful ways. Phase three involves dialogue to assist the conversation to endure past the time limit and translates it into people's lives outside of the contact. While this framework may seem quite linear, in practice it's much more rhizomatic with offshoots, detours, runs and perches, stop offs and back steps as we find our way together.

While the rites of passage metaphor characterizes the therapeutic conversation in stages or phases, I want to highlight that this linear representation is not, nor intended to be the full picture. The brief narrative single session is characterized in this way to separate from psychological characterizations and to share and emphasize some of the micro-skills. I do not mean to imply the reincorporation phase is an "ending" in the sense that someone has fully arrived at a revised identity or some sort of solution to their problem.

The single session conversation is not inseparable from the ongoing unfolding process of life. It is a "moment" in the ongoing process of becoming.[1] Said another way, it is likened to a momentary pause in an unfolding wave in the ocean. These conversations ripple out into life; a life that is continually becoming. Remember we had talked about the single session as like tipping the first domino or beginning to role a snowball down a hill. It is process, not a curative endpoint.

Further, but not to get too far from the topic at hand, we can bring into question the linear chronological unidirectional notion of time that tells us this happened and then that happened and then this happened next. It may be down the road that a sense of history is revised, looked at in a different way, influenced by reflection on something talked about in our single session days or years before. The conversation may germinate, so to speak, at a later date, collapsing time within the ongoing process of becoming. This places the concept of time in a more perspectival, interpretational, and cultural framework. As such, "time" is a device or a way of characterizing experiences by ordering them into a past, near now, and future orientation. This is important to brief narrative single session conversations highlighting time as a concept for meaning making. As noted in Chapter 2, past meanings can be revised influencing the near now and unfolding future. All this to say, there is always somewhere to go in these conversations, we are not bound by time, having to wait for internal developmental stages, or curative understandings of therapy.

The rites of passage metaphor serves as one useful representation of change as movement. There are other metaphors that also open possibility for these conversations. The notion of "seasons in life" lends itself well to brief narrative single session conversations. We can see people arrive in the winters of their life or, as Katherine May (2021) would refer to as "wintering". This is a time in life that's colder, less preferred, and demands some resilience. It often has required a time of preparation. Conversation assists people to embrace this more dormant time, and warm into renewed understandings. Progression is into the warmer summers as well as the inevitable cooling off of fall. In wintering, we assist people to weather the cold, persevere and re-emerge from the protection of hibernation. In this metaphor, life as cyclical is embraced as opposed to life as progress and normality favoured in Western culture. A fulsome exploration and application of this metaphor is beyond the scope of this chapter however, I wished to plant the seed that other metaphors are available and can help navigate these conversations. Chapters 5 through 7 will detail the three phases of the brief narrative single session further, but first let's give attention to what might be the most important accompanying skill.

Note

1 Vygotsky believed that people are always in a process of becoming as part of an ongoing social and cultural accomplishment achieved through interactions with the environment and with more skilled or knowledgeable individuals. It is a move away from the idea of development happening as an internal self-contained achievement. Development or growth is created by how we relate to each other. This is very relevant to single session conversations that take place within the social and cultural realms. Accepting the notion of "always becoming", possibility, hope and growth are highlighted.

References

Durrant, M. (1993). *Residential treatment: A cooperative, competency-based approach to therapy and program design*. New York: Norton.

Duvall, J. & Béres, L. (2007). Movement of identities: a map for therapeutic conversations about trauma. In C. Brown & T. Augusta-Scott (Eds.), *Narrative therapy: Making meaning, making lives* (pp. 229–250). California.

Duvall, J. & Béres, L. (2011). *Innovations in narrative therapy: Connecting practice, training, and research*. New York: W. W. Norton.

Hoyt, M. F. (2000). *Brief therapy and beyond: Stories, language, love and reality*. New York: W.W. Norton.

May, K. (2021). *Wintering: The power of rest and retreat in difficult times*. Cengage Gale.

Myerhoff, B. (1982). Life history among the elderly: Performance, visibility and re–membering. In Ruby, J. (ed): *A crack in the mirror. Reflective perspectives in anthropology*. Philadelphia: University of Pennsylvania Press.

Myerhoff, B. (1986). Life not death in Venice: Its second life. In V. Turner & E. Bruner (Eds.), *The Anthropology of Experience*. Chicago: University of Illinois Press.

Ray, W. A. & Keeney, B. (1993). *Resource focused therapy*. London: Karnac Books.

Sermijn, J. & Gergen, K. J. (2017). Spread the wings of your therapeutic potential: A reflecting process with Ken Gergen. *International Journal of Collaborative-Dialogic Practice*, 8(1), 57–68.

Shotter, J. (2009). Listening in a way that recognizes/realizes the world of 'the Other', *International Journal of Listening*, 23:1, 21–43, DOI: 10.1080/10904010802591904

Slive, A. & Bobele, M. (2011). *When one hour is all you have: Effective therapy for walk-in clients*. Phoenix, AZ: Zeig, Tucker, & Theisen.

Turner, V. W. (1969). *The ritual process: Structure and anti-structure*. Aldine Publishing Company.

Van Gennep, A. (1909). *The rites of passage*. Chicago: University of Chicago Press.

Van Gennep, A. (1960). *The rites of passage*. Chicago: University of Chicago Press.

White, M. (1995). *Re-authoring lives: Interviews & essays*. Adelaide, Australia: Dulwich Centre Publications.

White, M. (2000). Re-engaging with history: The absent but implicit. In M. White, *Reflections on narrative practice: Essays & interviews* (chapter 3, pp. 35–58). Adelaide: Dulwich Centre Publications.

White, M. (2011). *Narrative practice: Continuing the conversations*. New York: W.W. Norton.

White, M. & Epston, D. (1990). *Narrative means to therapeutic ends*. New York: W.W. Norton.

Chapter 4

Calibrating Your Brief Narrative Ear

Each tradition of therapeutic practice comes with ways of seeing and hearing participants, and ways of understanding distress and suffering. Whatever the encompassing lens, whether psychological, psychiatric, cognitive, systemic, or causal, our listening is limited. You can only see and hear what you train yourself to see and hear. Narrative therapy, informed by post-modern, post-structuralist, and constructionist ideas informs a particular practice of listening. It is this practice or as David Epson would call it, this species of listening that lends itself so well to the time constraint of single session therapy.

Anthropologist Victor Turner notes, "All expressions are radically plural" (1986, p.11) bringing our attention to a key understanding that informs our listening. People's expressions of life are not singular direct representations of experience, but rather expressions of meaning derived from an interpretation of those experiences. As such, any expression is linked to a multitude of alternate interpretations and meanings. There are multiple threads of meaning to an expression (Hibel & Polanco, 2010). Said another way, expressions are multi-layered. As such, multiple threads of meaning can be asked about and co-explored leading to novel conversation and new possibilities.

To hear the plurality in any expression, it is important to train our ear, so to speak, to be open to the many offshoots to possible meanings an expression links to. It requires an acute ear, calibrated to hear the smallest expression that can provide the start of a story-in-the-making. Given this, the kind of listening required is a skill that benefits from practice. That practice involves learning to listen for what an expression might suggest about people's experience of difference, diversity of daily life, and discernment between experiences past, near now, or dreamt in a future orientation.

Unordinary Difference

Difference is commonly thought of as a contradiction or binary such as problem/solution, right/wrong, functioning/non-functioning. However, to hear expressions as radically plural we are not listening in terms of ordinary difference. We

DOI: 10.4324/9781003431688-5

are not listening linearly for what's wrong in order to fix it. We are not listening for reasons for distress, insights into why the problem is happening or for symptoms of pathology. Those ways of listening in a time-constrained context risk closing down possibility.

Rather, we are listening for the swarms of alternate meanings connected to the expression. This is unordinary difference and encompasses all that material outside of the problem story across the timeline. "Our ears can be drawn to the ever-presentness of stories that are different from the problem story. Everything that is not the problem story becomes a possible site for the emergence of new meanings that can be ascribed more useful and more 'agentive' purpose'" (Carey, Walther & Russell, 2009, p. 322). We are listening to select from the meanings available that which may provide a starting point to the co-authoring of an alternative story (White & Epston, 1990), or what I refer to as a preferred story-in-the-making. This is listening with an intention to select material outside the dominant problem story to ask about and expand to co-craft alternative accounts (Hibel & Polanco, 2010).

The imagery of a rhizome has been adopted in narrative therapy (Walther & Carey, 2009; Reynolds & Polonco, 2012) to help orient us to unordinary difference and the plurality of expressions of life. Bamboo has a rhizomatic structure as well as strawberry plants and many of those pesky weeds that you try to pull up and the next thing you know you've traveled meters across your lawn following long filament roots that seem to go on endlessly. Adopting this structure, Deleuze and Guattari (1987) propose a rhizomatic understanding of thought as non-linear moving away from cause/effect linkages towards multiplicities that are connected. In contrast to common tree like structures representing hierarchy and linear linkages, the rhizome has no beginning or end but rather ever connecting offshoots to other appendages.

Adopting this imagery, we can imagine an expression of life connected to many alternate offshoots of meanings linked to and associated with other experiences that when followed can be brought into stories-in-the-making. "In relation to therapeutic practice we can consider how lines of rhizomatic inquiry can initiate off-shoots of stories which can then take root and develop as distinct but linked accounts of preferred story" (Walther & Carey, 2009 p. 5).

In practice then, when someone expresses, "I can't go on one more minute," we listen for the multitude of meanings connected to the statement that could provide the start of a story-in-the-making. You can imagine how in the pace of conversation this expression would race by us and become swallowed by the content of the problem story. However, with a brief narrative ear, in the moment of that expression, we can be listening for the swarm of unordinary difference connected to the overt statement and lying in the implied world of meaning such as:

- They are sharing that they are no longer okay with what is or has been happening.
- The expression can be seen as an action, movement away from those circumstances.
- To not be okay with what is happening means they must have a view of the life they want.
- To know the life they want, suggests they have experienced it at some point.
- They are continuing to carry on despite their circumstance.
- They have carried on to this point founded on a skillset or ability to cope.
- The act of carrying on speaks to an intention for their life.
- They are resisting what it is that has them questioning carrying on with life.

Listening for the multiplicity of meanings in this way shapes the kinds of questions we ask. We could respond with many questions that offshoot to potential storylines. What's happening that you are not okay with in your life? How have you gone on as long as you have? What picture of a different life have you held on to for so long? What does this distress suggest about what you want for your future? When was life more in harmony with how you would like it to be? What does it say about you that you have been able to carry on so long given what you are up against? Who in your life would not be surprised to know how you have been able to persevere? The responses to these sorts of questions could elicit a range of abilities, skills for living, and intentions for life that not only get onto a multi-storied life but provide a foundation for proposals for action that are more in harmony with the persons intentions and preferences for their life.

With a focus on "expressions of life" as our starting point of inquiry, we strive to resist imposing our own theoretical frames, categories, and pre-determined destinations for the conversation. "Expressions are the peoples' articulations, formulations, and representations of their own experience" (Bruner, 1986, p. 9). As the starting points for our inquiry, people's lived experience becomes the material for joint exploration and discovery, not hypothesized speculations by the professional. We are not replacing a story with a better story. We are co-crafting, weaving together, linking, and connecting preferred meanings structured by story, fabricated from people's own lived experiences and interpretations.

To orient to the complexity of this practice we will explore several categories of brief narrative listening. These categories are provided to aid in growing your listening skills, directing attention to the range of meanings within any expression.

The Principle of Double Listening

White (2000, 2003) outlines the principle of double listening to hear the plurality of meaning shared in any expression of distress. The practice of double listening orients us to recognize, hear, and honour a person's description of the problem story while simultaneously listening for material to shape the story-in-the-making. For instance, as we listen to the problem story, we are listening for what it speaks to about what is important to the person and what they want different. Listening doubly allows us to hear multiple entry points to possible stories-in-the-making. These entry points can be heard as concepts such as strengths, abilities, resilience, competence, skills for living, as well as implied hopes for life, wishes for things to be different, preferences for life and relationships, intentions, cherished values or beliefs, commitments, moral codes, and notions of preferred identity to name a few.

Why this is so important to single session and brief contexts is that double listening assists people to be doubly or multiply heard (White, 2000). For many, to not have an opportunity to share their concern would be unhelpful and off-putting. In the time we have together it is important to create space for the problem story fostering a sense of acknowledgement and understanding. Yet, it is equally important not to get stuck there. With careful listening and corresponding enquiry, we resist getting mired in a single storied account and enter multi-storied conversation. When we ask questions related to what the problem story speaks to about what matters to people and what they would like different they have an opportunity to enter into meaning making, exploring revised ideas about identity and possibility. We then have the opportunity to learn about their know-how and skills for living associated with what is emerging.

The principle of double listening provides the brief narrative therapist with an orientation to what we hear from people. It involves the understanding that any complaint is intimately linked to a vision of a preferred life. It is implied within the complaint.

Hearing What's Implied

To put into practice the principle of double listening is to listen for what is not said but implied within an expression. Listening for the absent but implicit involves the idea that we make meaning of any experience by contrasting it with some other experience(s) (White, 2003, 2006; Freedman, 2014). Inquiry relies on the appreciation that all problem descriptions are dependent on something contrasting, the un-stated out-of-focus background which renders the problem visible, the absent but implicit. For instance, to know "depression" means I must know the experience of "non-depression" otherwise I would not make sense of my experience as "depression". An expression is the visible side of this discernment and what it is in contrast to lies more in the background as implied material.

The unstated background material often relates to peoples' preferred experiences and/or important values and beliefs they hold. We can be on the lookout, listening for that implied background material, become curious about it, and assist it to the foreground through our inquiry. Further, we can then trace the hereditary[1] lines and history of that implied material. We can be curious as to where these values and beliefs have shown up in the distant past, recent past, and near now. How have they enacted them?

As an example, let's hear what the following expression of distress may speak to about the person's hopes for things to be different, values, beliefs, and intentions for life.

> Well, I have really bad mood swings from like anger. I get really obsessive around my boyfriend like I need to know where he is and who he's with when I'm not with him, so I end up calling him all the time or just sitting in my room crying. My old boyfriend cheated on me right in front of me at the semi-formal. That was one of the most horrible moments of my life. Then, when I go with my boyfriend now, his friends ignore me. It's like I'm not good enough for his friends.

If we double listen to this story, we certainly hear the expression of distress represented as mood swings, anger, the hurt from infidelity and being ignored. However, we simultaneously hear what's implied by that distress. The experience of anger may suggest certain values are being trespassed that are important. What might those values be, respect, independence, trust? We hear the distress related to being cheated on which implies this person must value and long for loyalty and trust in relationships otherwise being cheated on would not be a concern to them. We hear that they must have ideas about how people should treat each other, recognizing the recent treatment is not okay. This suggests they have more preferred relationships or have experienced them in the past. Listening in this way invites curiosity about what their distress might speak to about what is important to them, what they are seeking in relationships and what are red flags for them in relationships. This material, when brought into a storyline, may provide new ideas about steps to take to revise their relationships. They arrive at revised identity conclusions related to the distress. As opposed to being obsessive and not good enough, they may come to know their values more richly and how these values may show up in future relationships. It is through double listening to their distress for the absent but implicit[2] that these entry points come available.

Listening for Unique Outcomes

Out of the panorama of life experience very little tends to get storied. Infinite amounts of day to day, moment to moment information is filtered out to make life comprehendible. Much of it goes unnoticed, is not tended to, and as it travels to our biology it's converted and filtered further as the brain does its work. As a means to emphasize this idea, Gregory Bateson would start lectures with the question, "Can you see me?" He was stressing the idea that we can only see a representation of him assembled from the energy travelling throughout neurons and brain chemicals with any gaps being filled in during the processes. The point being, very little information gets tended to and what does forms a representative map not an exact duplication of the territory it refers to (Bateson, 1972). Events that do get storied, linked together, and ascribed meaning, themselves, are filtered with story serving as the map upon which they are placed. A great deal of information is left off the map.

One of the key roles of a brief narrative therapist is to listen for material left off the problem map. We listen for unique outcomes (White & Epston, 1990) and exceptions to the problem story. A unique outcome represents any event outside of or not predicted by the problem story. These acts of difference can be thoughts, feelings, actions, plans, beliefs, a desire, or commitment (Morgan, 2000). They may involve times when people have attempted to directly counter the problem, times when the influence of the problem was less severe/intense or when things were better. They can be heard in people's expressions such as, "I used to be in an abusive relationship..."; "I got so high but not as bad as other times..."; "Then I thought to myself, what if I have a good life...". Each of these expressions offers a meaningful offshoot to more preferred stories, whether it's knowing how to free themselves from relationships with abuse, movement away from a drug life, or countering thoughts of suicide.

In the pace of conversation these entry points come and go by very quickly. They are at risk of fading or going unnoticed unless we hear them and ask about them. They require that uncommon attentiveness to pick up on them and inquiry to hold them apart from the problem saturated story allowing for reflection. As we train our ear to pick up on acts of difference, we are able to craft and ask questions to elicit the details to begin co-crafting a more preferred account of life and identity.

Maggie Carey (2006), details further what we can listen for seeking unique outcomes. We can listen for:

- Descriptions of moving away from or towards something in life.
  "I don't want to go down that path anymore." "I'm sick and tired of this."
- Expressing a learning.
  "I know that there are certain things that are just not right for me.". "I get it, I just don't care.", "I realized that's not what I want for my children."
- Making a decision.
  "I'm not going to get involved in that stuff anymore.", "I swore I'd never be like my parents were with me", "These aren't people I want in my life anymore."

- Holding a position.
  "It's just not fair, that's not the ways it should be", "That's not how people should be treated."
  "I knew I needed help, it's just a matter of admitting it."
- Past tenses.
  "I didn't want to be here, I wanted to go…", "They used to be in trouble all the time…"

Each of these statements provides an entry point, as we can learn what someone is moving towards, what difference a learning will make, what values and intentions inform a decision, what a position says about what is important to a person, and what has changed as time has unfolded.

Hearing Expressions as Actions

Returning to therapy as a rite of passage, the first stage, separation, involves a time of preparation and movement away from the way things are and/or from unwelcome ideas of identity. For our purposes, when someone attends the session, that action of attendance marks the beginning of a transition. It represents a purposeful separation from the old ways of doing and viewing and implies a vision of a more preferred life. It marks a shift from one way of viewing oneself to another.

This idea shapes how we hear people's expressions of distress. If attending a single session and sharing about distress is understood as separation from a context and/or status that is no longer viable, than it is movement. It is an action! We can understand it as part of a broader unfolding life journey and be curious about what they are moving towards. We can be curious about what kind of action an expression of distress is.

In hearing expressions of distress as actions, we are again invoking Whites' concept of "the absent but implicit" (White, 2003). While the expression of distress is the visible, explicit part we hear, we can also listen for what is implied in that expression but not spoken overtly. What is implied by coming to therapy? What is implied by sharing distress? It implies the person's current situation and/or identity are no longer okay with them. To know it is no longer okay means they must have a picture or vision or hope for how they would like things to be different–some place they are moving towards. And last, to know of such a destination or preferred life means they likely have experienced that preferred life in some way already in some context or place.

We can be curious about what kind of action this is that people are taking. Could the expressions be an act of resistance, protest, questioning the way things are, refusal to go along with or be complicit with injustice? Is coming to therapy an act to reclaim aspects of life that have become absented, eroded, and overridden? Could the step represent efforts to renew ones hopes and dreams for their life? What might their vision of a preferred life be? Many questions come available within his metaphor. See Chapters 14 and 15 for a thorough sample of these questions as we hear expressions as action.

In meeting with a young man and his father I explored what his attendance suggested about his intentions for his life and relationship with family.

Scot:	Mike, I noticed in the paperwork that you really want this to be over quickly, is that correct?
Mike:	Yep, the sooner the better. I don't need therapy!
S:	Okay, yet you came today with your dad and your social worker and were willing to sit in?
M:	Ya, well, they think I need help still and I'm trying get along with my dad so...
S:	So you decided well I'll go and give it a try because I want to get along with my dad and... Can I ask a question about that?
M:	Sure fine.
S:	What do you think it says about what you want for your life given that you came today even though you didn't really want to, but did it anyway and especially for your dad?
M:	Well, we've been apart for two years now because I was in treatment, you know, for drugs and stuff so I want to have a dad and a life, you know.
S:	What you said really interests me Mike, can I ask a few more questions about that?
M:	Sure fine.
S:	So, coming today says that you want a life for yourself, and you want a dad in your life, when did you decide that? When did you come to say to yourself 'hey this is the future I want and I want to have people in my life, people that mean something to me like my dad?
M:	Well, I overdosed on drugs and, well, I survived so I decided to make some decisions about what I was doing.
S:	So that was like a turning point for you, was it?
M:	Ya, I guess it was!
S:	How's this conversation going for you so far, is it okay?
M:	Ya, I hadn't really talked about this stuff before, but this is good.
S:	Are you good to continue for a bit more?
M:	Ya sure, this is good.

This conversation could have begun in many ways and proceeded to many other offshoots of stories. However, by viewing Mike's attendance as an act of separation, I was curious about what it said about what he wanted for his life by coming to the walk-in. A story begins to emerge about a turning point in which he became clearer on what he wanted for his life. Mike's own curiosity begins to emerge about this and is reflected in his permission to carry on with the conversation.

Non-Structuralist Informed Listening

Within the principle of double listening, we can tune our ear to hear concepts specifically shaped by the influence of non-structural meta-theory. For the brief narrative therapist, the influence of non-structuralist ideas has contributed significantly to narrative practice expanding what we listen for and enquire about. White, (2006) summarizes concisely noting, "Through non-structuralist enquiries we become fascinated with the particularities of people's lives, their actions that are an expression of certain intentions, commitments, principles, hopes, dreams, passions, and beliefs" (p. 118). We listen understanding people's actions as clues to certain intentions for their life, hopes for things to be different, principles, or commitments to people and beliefs.

Young (2006, 2008) notes how this inquiry comes from a post-structuralist curiosity. That is a curiosity about what people's choices speak to about their intentions and what the values and beliefs are that those intentions are founded on or shaped by. Questions that arise from this style of listening assist story expansion.

I once worked with a 13-year-old youth who was suffering from ulcerative colitis. Stress would significantly increase his physical symptoms, and he had noted that one of his greatest stresses was his relationship with his father. He noted he feared his father who enforced strict rules. He had asked me to speak to his father about this. Meeting with him, I asked, "Did you know your boy was scared of you?"

His father's response was a firm, "Yes, so what?"

I said, "So you are okay with your son being scared of you?"

"Yes," was his reply.

At this juncture, a single-sided listening to this expression may invite us into judgment and increasing concern for what we are hearing. However, when guided by our curiosity and non-structural listening, that is, listening for intentions—we could ask, "Why are you okay with your boy being scared of you?"

"Because I know if my boy is scared of me, he won't be out drinking, drugging, and sexing around with all those other delinquents out there!"

Through a non-structuralist inquiry, we hear about how much this father loves and cares about his son and his son's safety. It is his intention to protect. When we hear this expression of protection, we can respond to it, assisting it to become better known as it is explored and shared.

"So it's important to you to keep your son safe?"

"Yes, of course."

"Well, suppose you could keep your son safe without him being scared of you, would you be open to that?"

"Of course, but nothing else works."

"Well, would it be useful to hear what I've heard other fathers try with some success?"

"Ya, I guess it wouldn't hurt."

Throughout my brief narrative single session conversations, asking about intentions has led out of many storylines of conflict and divide into loving stories-in-the-making.

Listening for Insider Knowledge

Concerning ourselves with people's expressions of life and stories, we become immersed in what they know and know how to do. We are interested in the little things, the details of people's ideas and practices, the ways they navigate life and their circumstances. It's that know-how that has been crafted through the rigor of day-to-day living that and can be canvased and brought to bear on the problem.

Listening for people's insider knowledge relies on a mindset which recognizes that people bring with them to these conversations a vast pool of knowledge that can be drawn from and languaged further into existence. Our role is to listen for and be curious about someone's knowledge inviting them to teach us about it. We want to learn as much as we can from them, writing their ideas in quotes, and referencing them as best as possible. People's lived experiences become points of entry to stories-in-the-making.

This is particularly useful and important to single session therapy as drawing from people's pool of know-how ensures it is context specific. Although it may often get discounted, is rarely spoken about or goes unnoticed, when asked about, it emerges, develops further, and can be utilized to address problematic circumstances. This differs greatly from the deployment of pre-determined concepts, strategies, or teachings that are more universally based.

As an example, a young person I met with found herself frozen in life with fear of the world. This fear was interfering with her school attendance, her ability to visit friends, and her sleep. However, in getting introduced to this young person, she shared a favourite summer memory with me of a family trip to the coast where she went jumping off a pier to swim in the ocean. Arrested by this circumstance, I shared my shock exclaiming, "You did what, jumped into the ocean?"

I continued, "Do you know what's in there? There are big fish with big teeth and weird-looking things."

Unswayed, she replied, "Yes, I know!"

To satisfy my curiosity, I followed with my efforts to invite her to mentor me in this ability. I inquired, "How did you do that then? How did you not let fear stop you from going into the ocean and that becoming one of your favorite memories?"

"It was fun, so I just did it," she explained.

"So, is fun a bit of an antidote to fear, do you suppose?"

She had supposed so. I continued, "Do you also guess you were using your courage a bit too, or all you needed was a bit of fun?"

She guessed she had used some courage as well. This led to an exciting conversation about the history of her courage as an antidote to fears that provided her with many ideas to go home with to try out. Inviting people to mentor us in their knowledge provides not only material for linking into stories-in-the-making but assists them to experience themselves as the knower.

Listening for Plot

In listening for plot, we are again double listening, tuning into the overarching theme of the problem story and sentiments counter to that theme. Listening in this way, "… in working to identify contradictions to the dominant plot, rather than seeking contradictions to the problem, we find a broad field of enquiry opening before us" (White, 1995, p.200). Plots may include life as futile, an overarching sense of helplessness, an account of personal failure, themes of being trapped, worthlessness, or understandings of identity as disordered to list a few. Hearing these themes, we can be on the look for and curious about material that counters the problem story theme. These are accounts of personal agency, hope, worth, and preferred identity.

As an example, I met with a person who had frequented the walk-in therapy clinic. They had seen a few different staff who each focused on the persons presenting complaint that they were experiencing low mood. Together, they generated strategies and ideas to try to lessen the problem, yet the person continued to return noting no progress. This was somewhat perplexing for staff who had thought their single sessions were useful as at the time the person had given that feedback.

Given this, I made an effort to listen to the description of the problem but to also zoom out and listen for the theme of the problem story. What emerged was an overarching view from the participant that their distress was their "curse" in a sense. It was something the world cast upon them, around their whole life, and part of just how their life is. This plot line of a sense of helplessness and resignation to outside forces helped to shape a very different kind of conversation.

We discussed the curse and the details of its effects. What events did he view as curse related? Had the curse tried to take his hope from him? Had it tried to blind him from any progress in life? Had it invited him to forecast a future for himself of more of the same? He outlined some key moments from a difficult life he had led. This included growing up with a caregiver who used abuse and often forecast a very negative future for him.

Unmasking the meaning made of a difficult life seemed to assist him to reposition to the curse and we began to outline signs that the curse is lifting. What did it mean that the person had recently started a new job? What were the steps they had taken to make that happen even with a curse to bear? What did it suggest that he did not use abuse in his relationship with his children and that he refused to forecast a negative future for them? What did it mean that they remained in his life and wanted to spend time with him? Could the anti-curse have anything to do with his commitment to refuse to use abuse in relationships?

At the conclusion of our talk, he had noted how this was a very different kind of conversation than he had previously, and it was a different kind of useful. He left with a project to continue to lift the curse.

Listening Knowing Identity is Relationally Shaped

As interpretive beings, people draw conclusions about who they are from their interactions and life events. Negative identity conclusions can come to represent the totality of a person, limiting the ways they respond to life. In understanding identity as fluid and relational, we can listen for preferred identity and developments that align more with that preferred way of seeing oneself. This assists us to keep present the identity project we are engaged in and to support storylines that rehabilitate limiting negative identity conclusions.

We hear these conclusions as people identify themselves through a diagnosis such as "I'm Bipolar". We hear negative conclusions such as "I can't do anything right, or I'm unlovable". These expressions are clues to us about the oppressive story of identity, prompting conversations to get on to more preferred accounts of identity.

A mother I had met with described her long held understanding of *worthlessness* as she had struggled to raise her children through the ups and downs of a drug life. However, following a very dark time of isolation and despair, she had decided to visit her doctor, restart medication, and reclaim her sleep. She named these actions "self-care steps" and upon further enquiry began to link them to a growing sense of *self-worth* she was experiencing within new and safe relationships. It was through listening for the overarching plot and knowing identity is not fixed but relationally shaped that this emerging identity became possible.

Listening to Problems as Separate from People

Founded on the assumption the person is the person and the problem is the problem, listening as though problems are separate from people aids in facilitating externalizing conversations. We are on the lookout for the ways people are oppressed by the problem and the tactics and tricks the problem uses to recruit people. We hear the ideas problems try to have people believe about themselves, their relationships and the world in general.

Listening as though problems are separate from people, we can also notice and hear the ways people resist problems in their daily lives. We can listen for times when the problems' oppression is incomplete. We can pick up on peoples' acts of resistance through counter thoughts/ feelings/ actions that provide the story fragments to be developed into a counter-story and stories of personal agency. Listening in this way, it can help to picture the problem as an external entity acting upon the person, using tactics and tricks to recruit them, and telling lies or exaggerations as a means to limit possibility. We'll revisit this kind of listening more thoroughly in Chapter 10 as we discuss externalizing conversations in single session therapy.

The commonality in all these ways of listening is the primary interest in the experience and understandings of the other. Out of all the skills I teach, listening in this way seems to be the most difficult for therapists to learn and sustain. I think being inundated with models that narrow the field of interest to fit their framework has an effect on therapists. The listening in a brief narrative therapy requires an intentional separation from model informed listening. David Epston has referenced it as a species of listening informed by ethnographic imagination (Epston, 2001). This is an ability to embrace curiosity and question one's own and one's own cultural understandings of life. He writes,

> It requires a different sort of inquiry, one that involves setting to one side one's own assumptions, making no pretences that you can know another's experience and 'walk in their shoes', but rather entering into an inquiry based on ethnographic imagination, whereby you seek their versions of how they go about the living of their lives.

David situates this listening within the position of co-researching with those who consult us. Together with participants, we are co-researching problems and the very particular alternative knowledges that people have crafted in order to address them. This positioning is well suited to SST, assisting us to resist colonizing people into de-contextual models of therapy. As a co-researcher we assist in archiving the emerging knowledge in a way that it is there for people when they need it and can be shared with others to assist them. In a brief narrative practice this finds circulation through various take-away and leave-behind documents which we will explore in Chapters 8 and 9.

In this chapter, I have outlined the kinds of listening favourable to brief narrative single session conversations. Recognizing all expressions are radically plural, we are listening with intention, for ideas or events that might have otherwise been neglected and can be brought forward in a spirit of co-research. As Riikonen (in Malinen, 2001, p. 215) points out, these promising developments are like sparks or butterflies as it takes great watchfulness and uncommon attentiveness to catch them. Informed by an uncommon understanding of difference, we are listening with intention and purpose to supply the activity of story development or story expansion. This skill requires great discipline and focus. Again, all that is not the problem story becomes a possible site for the start of a story-in-the-making. This is what is so favourable to single session and time constrained work.

Notes

1 David Epston has referred to tracing the hereditary lines as part of inquiries of genealogy within wonderfulness interviews that trace a moral virtue backwards through the generations to distant sources. The effect can be to foster a sense of connection across generations, breaking isolation and creating meaningful connections to family. (See Marsten, Epston & Markham, 2016, p. 40–45.)
2 White (2003) drew heavily from the work of French philosopher Jacque Derrida in describing the absent but implicit. Derrida described how all meanings are arrived at through a process of discernment from what they are not. These contrasting meanings are implied but not overtly stated. See Derrida, 1978; White, 2001. Michael's application of the absent but implicit, to me, is one of the most important and influential practices to emerge in the field.

References

Bateson, G. (1972). *Steps to an ecology of mind.* New York: Chandler.
Bruner, E. M. (1986). Experience and its expressions. In V. W. Turner & E. M. Bruner (Eds.), *The anthropology of experience* (pp. 3–30). University of Illinois Press.
Carey, M. (2006). *Narrative Therapy* [Workshop Handout].
Carey, M., Walther, S. & Russell, S. (2009). The absent but implicit: A map to support therapeutic enquiry. *Family Process, 48*(3), 319–331. https://doi.org/10.1111/j.1545-5300.2009.01285.x
Deleuze, G. & Guattari, F. (1987; published 1980). *A thousand plateaus: Capitalism and schizophrenia,* translated Brian Massumi. Minneapolis: University of Minnesota Press.
Derrida, J. (1978). *Writing and difference.* Chicago: University of Chicago Press.
Epston, D. (2001). Anthropology, archives, co-research and narrative therapy. In D. Denborough (Ed.), *Family therapy: Exploring the field's past, present and possible futures* (pp. 161–166). Dulwich Centre Publications.
Freedman, J. (2014). Witnessing and positioning: structuring narrative therapy with families and couples. *The International Journal of Narrative Therapy and Community Work, 1*(March), 1–4.
Hibel, J. & Polanco, M. (2010). Tuning the ear: Listening in narrative therapy. *Journal of Systemic Therapies* March, *29*(1), 51–66.
Malinen, T. (2001). On using appreciative language in constructing promising/illusionistic realities. *Australian and New Zealand Journal of Family Therapy, 22*(4).
Marsten, D., Epston, D. & Markham, L. (2016). *Narrative therapy in wonderland: Connecting with children's imaginative know-how.* New York: W. W. Norton & Company.

Morgan, A. (2000). *What is narrative therapy? An easy-to-read introduction.* Adelaide, Australia: Dulwich Centre Publications.

Reynolds, V. & Polanco, M. (2012). An ethical stance for justice-doing in community work and therapy. *Journal of Systemic Therapies. 31*(4), 18–33.

Turner, V. & Bruner, E. (Eds.). (1986). *The anthropology of experience.* Chicago: University of Illinois Press.

Walther, S. & Carey, M. (2009). Narrative therapy, difference and possibility: inviting new beginnings. *Context,* 3–8.

White, M. (1995). *Re-authoring lives: Interviews & essays.* Adelaide, Australia: Dulwich Centre Publications.

White, M. (2000). Re-engaging with history: The absent but implicit. In White, M.: *Reflections on narrative practice: Essays & interviews* (chapter 3, pp.35–58). Adelaide, Australia: Dulwich Centre Publications.

White, M. (2001). Folk psychology and narrative practice. *Dulwich Centre Journal,* (2), 1–37. Reprinted in M. White (2004). *Narrative practice and exotic lives: Resurrecting diversity in everyday life* (pp. 59–118). Adelaide, Australia: Dulwich Centre Publications.

White, M. (2003). Narrative Practice and community assignments. *International Journal of Narrative Therapy and Community Work, 2003*(2), 17–55.

White, M. & Epston, D. (1990). *Narrative means to therapeutic ends.* New York: W.W. Norton.

White, M. & Morgan, A. (2006). *Narrative therapy with children and their families.* Adelaide, Australia: Dulwich Centre Publications.

Young, K. (2006). *When all the time you have is now: Narrative practice at a walk-in therapy clinic.* Retrieved September 16, 2020, from Narrative Approaches website: https://narrativeapproaches.com/when-all-the-time-you-have-is-now-narrative-practice-at-a-walk-in-therapy-clinic/

Young, K. (2008). Narrative practice at a walk-in therapy clinic: Developing children's worry wisdom. *Journal of Systemic Therapies, 27*(4), 54–74.

Chapter 5

Phase One: Beginnings

In a single session therapy encounter, we therapists are aware of the choreography, but often the participants are not. Based on popular media representations of therapy, they come with preconceived ideas about what will happen. They may be nervous and begin with an introduction all about the problem. In other instances, they may be unclear about what they hope to accomplish, what is possible, or what they are supposed to do. Someone may have mandated their attendance, or they present multiple concerns to discuss.

Phase one provides a focus on how we begin our time and conversation together. Good beginnings make for better endings, meaning that how we convene and facilitate the start of the conversation will shape outcomes, including people's experience of the process. This phase directs our attention to the nuances of practice favourable to facilitating a useful single session.

Once again, I understand that attending a single session is an action signifying a person's separation from the way things are in their life, as they move towards a more preferred life. Given this, movement metaphors are fitting, and I can understand them as beginning a journey of sorts. As the host or senior partner in that moment, it's my responsibility to structure our time so that it is useful and safe. This chapter will focus on the beginning phase, including 1) pre-session paperwork, 2) structuring safety, 3) meeting people through stories of competency, 4) developing a focus for our time together, and 5) honouring the concern.

To me, the process begins as soon as a person or family comes in the door at the walk-in clinic. Our reception greets people and offers snacks and beverages to ensure they are not hungry. As many children and youth arrive after school, those snacks are popular. Reception will orient participants to the paperwork, assisting if needed. Our paperwork typically includes a consent to service outlining the conditions in which people's information would not remain private, such as when we would have to share information with outside agents to ensure safety.

People are also provided with a service information sheet, briefly orienting them to our agency and items such as where information is kept, for how long, as well as the complaint procedure should they not have a good experience.

DOI: 10.4324/9781003431688-6

Your agency or accrediting body often outlines these items. The key is to keep them brief and available for reference, so paperwork is not intimidating. We also include a brief document that expands on the personal health and privacy requirements. Lastly, participants are asked to complete a pre-session questionnaire to orient us to a few items. Interestingly, in post-session feedback, warm and friendly greetings by reception are mentioned often, including appreciation for the snacks. It is a reminder about how important every process is in contributing to a safe, welcoming, and useful experience for participants.

Pre-Session Questionnaire

The pre-session questionnaire is an important part of the walk-in experience. We recognize that completing paperwork is not exempt from shaping how people will experience the process. The questions asked are not neutral but rather invite people to research their experiences. Given this, questions within our paperwork are purposefully crafted to not only orient us to what participants are coming about, but to also have people recall stories of their competence and events that could have them experience themselves in preferred ways.

This is an idea I believe is overlooked in services that use lengthy pre-screening tools. It's important to realize those tools shape people's experiences, generate meaning, and can leave people experiencing distress and hopelessness. Further, pre-session paperwork or screening tools inadvertently shape the process of therapy, orienting the therapists' attention towards specific material and away from other material. For this reason, it is important that any single session pre-session questionaries be in harmony with the therapeutic process itself. For instance, within a brief narrative process, paperwork needs to seek insider knowledge, material for more preferred stories-in-the–making and assist people to experience personal agency.

We have experimented with many questions over the years, teasing out which seem to elicit the most useful information, align with our process, and remain short and simple so as not to create a barrier for families. Here are some of the key questions and our rational for them. Depending on the context of your clinic, you may want to add some not included in this list.

Identifying Information

Designing paperwork in harmony with our practice ethics first gathers information needed to meet our fields requirements and to screen for risks. We collect information such as name, addresses, age/birthdate, gender preference, doctor, and family members. We invite participants to check a box identifying active custody/access dispute, current risk to self or others or violence in relationship. If indicated, we are sure to check-in about these circumstances and collaborate to find the safest way to proceed. At times, this may involve not proceeding or involvement of a collateral service.

What's most important to talk about today?

Following identifying information, the paperwork seeks to learn from the participant what their understanding is about what would be most important to talk about on this day. Asking what's most important to talk about today elicits the most pressing concern in the present. Not only is the question orienting the participant to what is happening in the here and now, the meta-message is that we are seeing them as knowing themselves and their life the best. We are viewing them as capable of knowing what they need to discuss. It's also a question that helps to narrow the conversational territory and acquaint us with their view of the concern.

Reviewing the responses to these questions orients the therapist to what the participant wants out of the time together. Employing our double listening, we are also oriented to hopes and wishes for things to be different. For instance, a response that reads, "I have been cutting a lot and I don't want to feel so depressed" suggests a few things to the therapist. First, the person has experienced non-depression or less depression at some point contrasted to their current experience. Second, there has been an increase in cutting, which implies they have resisted that amount of cutting in the past. Third, the comment suggests a wish for things to be different. Double listening to the answers in this way, flags for the therapist material to be curious about. It also assists the therapist to not get demoralized at the outset when focused on the problem story.

When are things better – even a little bit?

Additional questions nudge the participants to pay attention to more preferred circumstances in their life. This question, pre-supposing there are times when things are better, invites the participant early on to think about and re-experience those times through recall. An answer such as "When I'm with my friends" provides several openings for the therapist to ask more about. It implies relationships are important to the person. Perhaps they know themselves in more preferred ways through those relationships. That short answer orients the therapist to a world away from the problem description to material that may contribute to a story-in-the-making.

If 10 is the best and 1 is the worst, how are things in your life today?

Point of reference questions provide a different format of answer which can be easier for some people. Assigning a self-anchored number to their current situation helps to establish a point of reference and quickly orients the therapist to difference and possibility. Suppose the answer stated is the number three. The therapist is drawn to what the person is currently doing/thinking that has them at a three rather than lower. This material can be asked about and brought to the foreground, possibly informing a later proposal for action. Even the answer zero tells us a great deal about the severity of the situation. It also orients us to ask about how they have prevented the situation from being in the minus category. Working this scale in session, we can learn about the best things have been, and what the person was doing differently at that time. Together, we can speculate about what they would be doing differently should they move up the scale even a little.

What would someone else like and respect most about you if they had a lot of time to get to know you? it's okay to guess!

This question and the following question from David Epston in Young (2006) have become popular generative questions in pre-session paperwork. Years ago, we started out asking people to please list their strengths with the idea that we could follow-up about these. However, typically we received one-word responses or no response at all. We then listed several strengths which in hindsight were very Western privileged and culturally narrow, but we asked people to circle all that apply. Again, we saw one circled or none. Moving to this question style elicited a far more detailed response. Adapted for parents and children, it reads: *If we had months or years to get to know your child, what would we come to know and appreciate about them?*

The purpose of these questions is to begin to orient a focus towards competence and/or their children's competence. Answers provide the therapist with possible entry points into preferred accounts of identity and life that could be researched and brought to address the problem.

What else would be important for us to know about your situation?

This question elicits the context within which the concern is experienced. Context is an important part of problem description. It helps to provide a frame in which to make sense of events and people's responses. It brings to light the circumstances that have the concern make sense. It foregrounds the experience of past or ongoing injustice or oppression or identifies relationships that may need addressing. You can imagine how answers such as "we are currently living in the women's shelter", or "I just left an abusive relationship", or "I was unfairly fired from my job and may lose my home", all provide important information contextualizing distress.

For us to be most useful, is there anything important for us to know about your culture, ethnicity, spirituality, language, sexual orientation, gender identity/expression, mental or physical health, or other?

Answers to this question speaks to the broader context of people's lives. This allows us, in a small way, to meet the person in context. Learning about this context early helps us to ask questions that contextualize the story-in-the-making within a broader historical frame. We can learn from participants what these aspects make possible for them, contribute to the life or perhaps how they create barriers. We can be curious about when they became connected to these aspects and who may have contributed to their place in their life. It helps us to learn about any potential barriers to service that need to be addressed.

With 10 being the best and 1 very poor, please rate your (your child's) quality of sleep

Most recently we have added a sleep rating question. This came about out of concern that children brought to the clinic were experiencing sleep problems. Many of these youth had been given a diagnosis of ADHD yet their sleep remained troublesome. Sleep problems have been linked to affecting the development of executive functioning (Turnbull, Reid & Morton, 2013). With the addition of this question an important contextual aspect remains more present for our team.

Once completed, the paperwork is briefly reviewed by our team to discern possible entry points to be explored and to match a therapist considering the presenting concern and therapist's specific skill set. The therapist then greets and brings the participants into the meeting space to begin. Appendices 1 and 2 provide sample pre-session questionnaires for walk-in therapy. Again, the spirit of these questions is to nudge people towards the recall of their competence and times more preferred. This is founded on the understanding that questions are creational, influential and generate experience.

We are not engaging in traditional problem assessment or using universal tools to screen for problems, to assist with prioritizing distribution of services to those viewed most at risk, or to gather information for data-informed planning. Insoo Kim Berg, the co-founder of solution-focused brief therapy used to say that information is only as useful as it relates to what people want different. In SST with the focus on difference, possibility, and the future, we want to get people to the service as quickly as possible and orient them towards difference each step along the way.

Structuring Safety

Structuring safety refers to the practices of "… negotiating or co-constructing the conditions, structures and agreements that will make space for safe-enough work alongside [people]" (Richardson/Kianewesquao & Reynolds, 2014 p. 151). This involves intentional practices that help people to know what is to come and invites their permission to begin the conversation. Structuring safety requires an understanding of the complexities of power and work within an anti-oppressive framework (p.151). In beginning these conversations, I seek to start from a safe enough place. It's important to me that the participant(s) experience comfort, privacy, and have a sense of what to expect from the process.

First, in the same way you might welcome a guest to your home, I welcome people and provide a short tour of the venue orienting to the washrooms and our meeting space. I ensure they are okay with our meeting space, as at times space can remind people of other places in which they had to give testimony or report abuses. I ask permission to close the door, so people don't overhear or interrupt us. Understandably, some children and youth prefer the door open. Once settled into the space, children will often want to explore a bit. I then take some time to check in briefly about whether people understood the consent to service presented in the waiting room and our responsibility to involve others in the conversation should safety be at risk.

> Did you have a chance to review the consent to service or have any questions about it? Just to briefly review, our conversation is private. It stays with us but there are some times that we may have to bring other people into the conversation, especially should we believe safety is compromised.

The phrasing "we may have to bring other people into the conversation" is purposefully different from "duty to report". This is to position collaboratively and set the scene for whoever becomes involved to work together should that be needed. I then canvas permission to orient them to our time together following a brief introduction of myself.

> Would it be okay if I introduce myself so I'm not a total stranger and perhaps share a bit about the walk-in/single session process and then we can get on to what would be important to talk about today?

I locate myself sharing some personal and professional information. Personal information may include my interests and hobbies to help melt the unspoken power relation the context creates. Locating myself professionally, I share how long I've been meeting with families and say a bit about my style in these conversations. This was common practice for Michael White during training consultations.

A Preamble

Following my welcoming I note:

> I see the time we have together as a chance to have a conversation and my hope is that it's useful in some way. You[1] may find it's all you need and leave with a different way of looking at things or perhaps some ideas about steps to try out and practice afterwards. However, there are no guarantees, so should you not find this useful please let me know.

The preamble serves the following purposes:

- In noting that this is a chance to have a "conversation", I'm setting the stage for dialogue. This is an intentional phrase inviting people to enter into something familiar and perhaps different from their preconceived notion of what a "therapeutic conversation" is.
- I also note my hope is that it is a "useful" conversation. The word "useful" is chosen in contrast to the word "helpful". My intention is for the conversation to be useful. The meta-message to the family is that they can choose to "use" what is offered or not. I view them as knowledgeable about their own life and able to choose what will fit for them. They have the control and I know them in this way. The phrase helpful risks positioning me as the knower, possessing something they don't, and as the one doing the work.
- In highlighting the hope for the *conversation* to be useful, I am de-centering myself as the agent of change. Implying the conversation will be useful whether it is with me, or another walk-in therapist resists inadvertently fostering reliance on me as the service provider. My hope is for people to develop a relationship to the service rather than to me. That way they would not hesitate to come back and meet with any of the service providers.
- To suggest "you will leave here with a new/different way of looking at things or an idea to try out and practice when you return home" opens the field of possibility but also sends implicit messages about the process and outcome of the conversation. It seeds positive expectation and the notion that there are multiple ways to look at situations, predicaments, and concerns. It seeds the notion that they may be required to engage in action following the conversation, so our conversation is a starting point in the process. This journey will require practice in the real world.
- It is important to note that there are "no guarantees" that the single session will make any difference to their situation in order to inoculate against the

misattribution of personal failure. Many people arrive with the idea that the therapist will know what to do or fix them or their child. We strive to lower that expectation so that if they return home and the difficulties persist, they don't story their experience as personal failure. We want to suggest there are no guarantees and should things continue to be difficult after the session, it is to be expected at times. If the session proves not useful it is okay to return to the walk-in to continue the conversation and rework or revise the plan of action.

Continuing to structure safety, I go over what to expect from the single session. I want participants to know what information I am asking about, collecting, and where that information gets archived.

> I tend to ask a lot of questions. If I ask a question that makes little sense or I don't have business asking, can you please let me know? Also, would it be okay if I take some notes as we go because it helps me remember things and there are some things that we might want to come back to? I'll do my best to get your words down, not my words, and one thing we do here at the walk-in is to make a copy of this note for you, so you have a copy for yourself if you want. Do you have any questions for me or about this process?

After setting the stage for our conversation and tending to structuring safety, the focus shifts to the world of the participant.

Meeting People Through Stories of Competence and Preferred Identity

Many traditions of therapeutic practice would have people introduced through the telling of the problem. Children are particularly vulnerable to this introduction by their care givers. Imagine through a child's eyes being introduced as attention deficit or disordered. A problem focused introduction risks distancing a person from the conversation and affects the growing relationship with the service provider. To inoculate against such risk, we purposefully break away from therapeutic conversational tendencies that meet people through the telling of the problem. This involves a concerted effort to begin the session by getting to know people through stories of competence and preferred identity.

If I was meeting with children and parents, I first meet the child as they are likely the most marginal voice in the room. My intention is to make space for an introduction through stories of their competence and times of preferred identity. I often start by asking their permission to get to know them through their parent.

> I imagine no one likes to be introduced through the telling of their problems, so I wonder if it would be okay for me to get to know you through

your parents' loving eyes and hear what it is they have come to appreciate about you?

I'm wondering if a nice way to meet you today would be to hear from your mom about what it is that she brags to the other moms about you?

If I were meeting with a couple, I might ask:

Before we come to your concerns, can I first hear about what drew you two together in the beginning? What have you come to know and appreciate about each other over your time together?

If I were meeting a family:

Okay, who here is the funniest, cooks the best, or is best at video games?

Through these questions, we learn about attributes, interests, hobbies, and the abilities that they may come to use to shape their lives in more preferred ways. In meeting people this way, early in the conversation, we foreground what people bring to the process that may be put to agentive use to address their circumstances. Further, we may hear about other identity stories unrelated to the problem description. We hear how people are athletes, artists, and supervisors, hardworking, generous, a big sister or brother. All these elements that are presented outside of the problem description offer, very early on in the single session conversation, entry points into possibility.

It is rare but occasionally a caregiver may struggle to come up with something they love, appreciate or like about their child or a spouse will struggle to share something appreciated about their partner. This speaks to how widely the problem has blinded the caregiver or spouse. It's a sign of how dominant the problem story has become. However, I do not leave someone to struggle to answer this or without answering. I would use a follow-up question such as:

I don't imagine things have always been as difficult as they seem now, tell me a story about a time when you had some fun together or a loving moment?

I could also editorialize and then engage speculation.

Again, I'll come to what brings you in shortly, but I don't imagine anyone wants to be introduced through the telling of the problems in their life so I'm just wondering for instance what is it the two of you like to do together or do you have a shared favourite movie or music? Do you have pets or hobbies?

There is always a glimmer of common ground or a preferred moment of shared time that we can draw upon as an entry point into a story of competence. With any answer, I can begin weaving back and forth asking questions that draw out and link together preferred times.

- Well, who tells the best jokes in the family?
- Who is the best cook?
- What's a favourite tv show you enjoy?

These simple questions quickly open doors to more preferred times and further questions.

- So, is a sense of humour important to you? Who do you suppose you learned that from? (Turning to a family member) Tell me about a time they cracked you up?
- What's a favourite meal you remember they cooked? How come that was a favourite? (Turning to the family member) Did you know that was their favourite? What's it like to know they enjoy your cooking? It that something you hope to pass on to them one day?

Bringing further intention and structure to this process, David Epston (in Marsten, D., Epston, D., & Markham, L., 2016) has outlined what he refers to as "wonderfulness interviewing".[2] He highlights a very specific way to meet people away from the problem. This practice puts the assumption "The problem is the problem, the person is the person" into action. He highlights prefacing a transition to this conversation by asking the participant if it would be okay to get to know them away from the problem, whatever it might be. I believe this prefacing is important to assist people to transition to this kind of conversation. I will often add my reasoning for asking to meet them this way to seed that this is not idle chat, but purposeful.

> Before we come to the problem that you are here about, whatever it might be, I'm wondering if I could get to know you though some stories away from the problem first? The reason is that I imagine there's a great deal of your life lived away from the problem and I'm hoping to learn about what you might have to put up against this problem. Is that okay?

Epston would then seek to hear about a storied example of their wonderful-nesses. Asking people to share a story about where that competency has shown up in life moves away from gathering a laundry list of compliments to more meaningful tellings tied to storied examples of preferred identity.

> Can you tell me a story about where you really noticed that?
> Can you tell me a story about that to help me understand it more fully?

Proceeding through the genre of externalizing, the participant is invited to introduce the Problem to the Wonderfulnesses and confront the problem establishing an antagonist/protagonist relationship.

Whatever the problem is, do you think it knows about...?

Are you okay with this problem in your life?

Suppose you were to introduce the problem to your determination what effects will that have on the Problem?

Through this inquiry, we become acquainted with what people have to put up against the problems in their lives. When the constellation of skills associated with interests and/or the knowledges and skills for living one employs become visible, we can quickly bring them to bear upon the problem to assist the person to alter their relationship with it. Within this inquiry, we meet people through identity stories that are more preferred and speak to their abilities to shape and direct their lives. Epston points out how these conversations can be restorative of people's dignity and the sense that they can make good decisions for themselves.

Most often, stories of exceptions, unique outcomes, and initiatives come forward when meeting people this way. The details of those events, when woven into stories-in-the-making, often contribute to the action plans crafted near the end of the session. They often contribute to the most useful action plans as the ideas build off of what people already know how to do.

Sample questions from Freeman, Epston & Lobovits, 1997.

To adults:

If there was something you could do every day forever, what would it be?

If I had years or months to get to know you, what do you imagine I'd come to appreciate about you?

What would your best friend note that they have come to know and admire about you through your friendship?

What should I know your partner has going for them to put up against the problem, whatever it might be?

What would I come to admire about your partner if I had months or years to get to know them? What is it that they've got to put up against this problem?

What can you tell me about your father/son relationship that stands apart from the problem?

What are your hopes and dreams for your partners future?

What are you all hoping to return to doing with him when the problems out of the way?

Inquiry from children's point of view:
What would your children say they appreciate most about you?
What are some of the things you have enjoyed doing together?
What do you imagine they brag to their friends about, about you?

Specific to parents:
At your proudest moment as a father/mother, what were you most proud of?
If I were a fly on the wall of your daughters everyday life, what would I admire
    about her that only those who live with her could possibly know?
What aspects of your son would you like me to know that make you feel you are
    a great mother/father?

Listen for the Themes

As we listen to people's responses to these questions, we are listening not only
for their skills, abilities and interests etc. but also for emerging themes to explore
further. Within these themes are storylines of competence in contrast to the
problem. We listen for:

- Answers involving problem solving.
  Likes video games, Enjoys puzzles.
- Answers valuing relationships.
  *Likes to hang out with friends, does babysitting, really close to her
  grandparents.*
- Answers related to preferred identity.
  *Smart for their age, an old soul, a really good person, really good at
  their job.*
- Answers highlighting adventure.
  Loves to go motorbiking, mountain climbing, paintball.
- Answers related to self-care and coping.
  *I like chill'n and watching Netflix, I'm a homebody; just me and my dog,
  Exercise; I like to walk and enjoy nature…*

These themes are clues to broader preferred identity stories that can be named,
explored, and rendered more visible and meaningful as the conversation
unfolds.

Developing Focus/Narrow the Conversational Territory

Narrative therapy has drawn on geographic concepts and imagery to talk about
meaning making in therapeutic conversations. Adopting geographic metaphors,
the conversation becomes a journey moving from known and familiar meanings

to what's possible to know and do (White, 2007). Meaning making becomes exploration in this space, across terrains, landscapes of the mind and galaxies of possibility. The conversational territory available for exploration is a vast, undiscovered terrain. Within a single session, it would not be possible to explore all experiences and meaning involved; the territory would be too large. We must set a course and narrow the conversational territory in a way that the meaning making journey remains relevant and useful to the participant, addressing what they came for.

On the other hand, we don't want to narrow the conversational territory to the extent that it limits possibility and novel ways to make sense of experience. That has been my concern with the Western notion of goal setting. The Western world is very goal focused. You are to move life forward, progress, gain resources and the way to do this is to set goals and achieve them. This thought has infiltrated therapeutic practice, making goal setting a prominent and often mandated feature of therapeutic conversation. While well intended, goal setting can introduce some hazards in single session therapy.

One hazard may be that in setting a goal for the session, the conversation is narrowed to such an extent that the range of options for change become limited. In ongoing service, we can revisit often, and revise goals as needed. However, in SST, you may not see the person again to make adjustments. A set goal can be taken up in an achieve/don't achieve, pass/fail understanding. This risks participants experiencing a sense of personal failure should they not meet their goal following the session. Further, goal pursuit may contribute to conversations locating the problem solely within an individual, asserting that the individual needs to change, making invisible contexts of injustice and oppression. For instance, the decontextualized goal of managing anger may make invisible the mistreatment someone experiences, to which they respond with anger. The goal of better mood may conceal the context of domestic violence. There is context to all problems, so context is often an important part of brief narrative conversations.

Given the vast possibilities for these encounters, early in the conversation, I seek to learn from the participant(s) what is most important to talk about and address given the time we have together. This is a means to narrow that conversational territory without setting a fixed destination. It's a way to set the focus for our time together. I can transition to this in many ways.

- What would be most important for us to talk about today?
- I notice from the paperwork that your hope was to not feel so depressed. Is this what you would like to focus on today?
- What are your hopes for this conversation given the time we have?
- (To parent) I noticed you wanted to talk about your child's ADHD. Is this right?
- (To child) Your parents were hoping to talk about ADHD today. Can I ask you what you think would be most important for us to talk about today?

In asking the participant about what to focus on, I am inviting them to prioritize and set the course for the conversation. This is important as within the time constraint of a single session, we want to be sure people get out of the time what they came for. Inviting a focus early on, ensuring to address that focus in the conversation and returning to reference it within a re-telling in phase three keeps the session on track and useful. The meta-message to the participants is that we are seeing them as most knowledgeable about their lives and capable of setting the most useful focus for the conversation.

Sometimes people share multiple concerns. It is important to narrow multiple concerns to one that is most pressing and may influence the others.

- So out of a, b, c, or d, which would be the most important for us to talk about today that might even influence the other concerns?
- Out of a, b, or c, which would be most useful to focus on give the time we have?

Sometimes people are sent by others. In those situations, we can elicit the referrers hopes for the conversation.

> Whose idea was it to come in today? (Probation) Okay, what's your guess about what your service provider was hoping we would talk about? Are you okay if I ask a few questions about that, or is there something else you'd like to focus on today?

With a set focus, it is important to check-in throughout the session to ensure we are continuing to talk about what is most important to the participant. This serves to keep the conversation on track throughout the encounter. We will refer back to the stated agreed upon focus in phase three to draw coherence to the session and contribute to a perception of difference and progress. As the conversation unfolds, by keeping the focus in mind, the therapist ensures people will get what they want out of our time together. There may be conversational detours along the way, but a focus assists us to stay relevant and helps the therapist resist getting lost in content.

Honouring the Account of the Problem

People naturally situate their experiences into stories about themselves and their lives (Bruner, 1990; White & Epston, 1990). In this phase, there is space for the participant to share the most significant story they are concerned about. It is a time to hear and honour the problem story and to hear about the other meaningful characters in their life connected to the story.

In the telling of the problem story, the multi-storied lives of people emerge. It is through careful double listening (White, 2000) and post-structuralist curiosity (Young, 2006) that we hear about aspects that can be discussed more thoroughly in phase two of our encounter. As noted in Chapter 4, we are listening for expressions[3] that serve as entry points into more preferred stories. As noted in Chapter 2, entry points are represented by concepts such as unique outcomes, exceptions to the problem, past initiatives, hopes, values, intentions, commitments, strengths, competencies, abilities, skills for living, and moral codes. Entry points may be found in externalizing conversations, listening for what is implied, and generally in any expression of preferred difference. All this material can provide a foundation for story expansion and future plans.

Other times, we may need to leave more space for the problem story. This speaks to watching the pace of the conversation, ensuring we honour people's distress yet remain active and tend to material that may inform stories-in-the-making. The movement back and forth, in and out of, across the telling of the problem and preferred events, is a weave of sorts. It's most often not a linear path but rhizomatic with offshoots from the problem to sprouts of possibility and difference. That's what makes these conversations so exciting as the destination is not yet known and together, we can arrive at unexpected, nourishing understandings of life's events.

Movement Metaphors

The rite of passage underscores change as movement. In every single session conversation, as early as possible, I try to inject the idea that in attending, the participant is embarking on a journey or beginning a life project (Freedman et al., 2002) of sort. The meeting is likened to taking a step on a longer journey. This involves the linguistic introduction of the metaphor through a short summary, such as

> So, this is like a journey you have been embarking on, taking steps along the way to free your life from the worries and what they have prevented you from enjoying each day?

The purpose of this is threefold:

- It implies that people have been taking steps and actions to address their circumstances long before they came to services. Often, these steps go unnoticed. By referring to them as "early steps" on a longer journey, they are more likely to be taken into a storyline that allies with their preferences.
- In noticing that they have already taken some steps counter to the problem, people may experience greater hope. This is the sense that they can take action in the face of distress and that they have a sense of what actions to take.
- The journey metaphor implies future steps and proposals for action later on, down the path, further on the journey will be required. It sets a pre-context for future steps and actions following the single session.

This chapter has drawn attention to the micro practices of the first phase of brief narrative single session therapy. As a place in which people are taking a step, separating from contexts and ways of seeing themselves that are no longer okay with them, how we begin these conversations matters. Narrowing the conversational territory and meeting people specifically through stories of competence helps to set a course that is useful and safe. Exercising our brief narrative ear, we tend to expressions that serve as entry points to preferred stories and ready us for the project of meaning generation and story expansion focused on in phase two.

Notes

1 This has often been phrased as "Many people find a single session is all they need…". The intention is to positively seed that it is a possibility that the person may only need one session. I do not use that phrasing out of concern that someone who doesn't find it useful like 'many others' may experience being marginalized or unintentionally othered. Positive seeding is important so I tend to use "you may…" instead.
2 David Epston provides a Wonderfulness Interview Guide in the chapter In Pursuit of Children's Virtues in Marsten, Epston, Markham (2016).
3 Edward Bruner in his introduction for *The Anthropology of Experience* highlights how often the unit of investigation is shaped by an imposed category derived from the authorities own ever-shifting theoretical frame. However, by focusing on narrative or any other expression of life, we leave the definition of the unit of investigation up to the people. Expressions of life are our entry points to meaning making. They are the "…peoples' articulations, formulations, and representations of their own experience" (Bruner, 1986, p.9). Important to SST, with a focus on people's expressions we are resisting inducting people into models of therapy that cannot be checked through future sessions for the effects on the person's life.

References

Bruner, E. M. (1986). Experience and its expressions. In V. W. Turner & E. M. Bruner (Eds.), *The anthropology of experience* (pp. 3–30). University of Illinois Press.

Bruner, J. (1990). *Acts of meaning.* Harvard University Press.

Freedman, J. & Combs, G. (2002). *Narrative therapy with couples… and a whole lot more! A collection of papers, essays and exercises.* Adelaide: Dulwich Centre Publications.

Freeman, J., Epston, D. & Lobovits, D. (1997). *Playful approaches to serious problems: Narrative therapy with children and their families.* New York: W.W. Norton.

Richardson, C. & Reynolds, V. (2014). Structuring safety in therapeutic work alongside indigenous survivors of residential schools. *The Canadian Journal of Native Studies, 34*(2), 147–164.

Turnbull, K., Reid, G.J. & Morton, J.B. (2013). Behavioral sleep problems and their potential impact on developing executive function in children. *Sleep, 36*(7), 1077–1084. http://dx.doi.org/10.5665/sleep.2814.

White, M. (2000). Re-engaging with history: The absent but implicit. In M. White, *Reflections on narrative practice: Essays & interviews* (chapter 3, pp. 35–58). Adelaide: Dulwich Centre Publications.

White, M. (2007). *Maps of narrative practice*. New York: W.W. Norton,.

White, M. & Epston, D. (1990). *Narrative means to therapeutic ends*. New York: W.W. Norton.

Young, K. (2006). *When all the time you have is now: Narrative practice at a walk-in therapy clinic*. Retrieved September 16, 2020, from Narrative Approaches website: https://narrativeapproaches.com/when-all-the-time-you-have-is-now-narrative-practice-at-a-walk-in-therapy-clinic/

Chapter 6

Phase Two: Meaning Generation and Story Expansion

Within the rites of passage metaphor, phase two is described as a liminal space, a space between destinations. We all experience liminality in life having to traverse physical settings. Hallways, sailing the open water, or parking lots serve as liminal places. They are spaces of transition leading to new destinations.

We also experience liminality in the many transitions of life. Marriage ceremony represents a transition from an autonomous life to a life in union. A relationship breakup can leave people searching to figure out who they are on their own. The loss of a loved one can leave us in an unfamiliar place, coping with grief. All these experiences mark transitions in life from one state to another. As noted previously, imagine the space and time for a trapeze performer between letting go and catching again.

Characterized by unfamiliar circumstance, the liminal space can be experienced as unsettling or confusing as people are trying to find their way and figure things out. It can be a time of struggle and hard work to navigate these spaces. Within the liminal phase, how people know themselves becomes increasingly ambiguous. They are separating from old ways of seeing themselves yet have not arrived at a more preferred identity.

Others may experience the liminal phase as exciting and freeing as they have time to engage in self-reflection and experiment with new ways of being in the world. The liminal period becomes a generative time, opening new opportunities and calling forth creativity. It's this generative aspect of the liminal space that lends itself so well to single session therapy.

In therapy, thinking of this middle part of the conversation as a liminal space orients us to a time for meaning making, re-storying, re-imagining, and revision. This is a generative time in the conversation. It provides a place to co-research problems and alternative knowledge and to talk about experiences in novel ways. It is a time to sift and sort, to figure out and explore who one is becoming. People can experience themselves in new ways.

Our questions assist people in the liminal space to find their way. They engage people in meaning making, assisting to explore, consider new or revised meanings, and expand those meanings. In this space, we understand meanings as

DOI: 10.4324/9781003431688-7

tentative, experimental, learning material, suggestive of what might be, and hinting at a revised notion of identity. This space is a place for exploration and discovery of what people know and know how to do. It is a time of linking and connecting through wonder and imagination.

Together, we are trying to find our way towards more preferred understandings about life and self. This positions us as co-travelers, each bringing something to the journey. The participant outlines the territory, and we bring some maps and a safe process to help navigate. This is an active time in the conversation as we ask many questions.

In entering an unfamiliar place, we can expect it to be difficult to separate from problem stories. Well circulated dominant narratives can eclipse or render insignificant information outside their plot. They are sticky and difficult to dislodge, liken to the burs that snag your clothes when walking in a field. Yet the struggle in this phase can lead to excitement and renewal as new discoveries are made and new possibilities come to light. I liken this phase and the revision of identity to trying on a new pair of shoes. While more stylish, they start out somewhat uncomfortable, but one day, once walked in, provide a comfortable fit.

In this middle phase conversation is likened to a boat entering the open water away from the stability of the dock and harbour. To get to the next destination, some navigation is needed. Within phase two, our concern is to assist people across the gap between the experience of the problem towards possibility and difference. This is important in single session work, as it is our responsibility to assist people to get somewhere in these conversations. Especially given the time constraint, we want to arrive somewhere more preferred by the end.

Navigating this phase is aided by the re-authoring process (White & Epston, 1990; White, 2007). Re-authoring helps people identify and link preferred events in their lives into stories. This involves much more than highlighting people's strength, pointing out positives, or listing what they can do. Linking preferred events into storylines assists the emerging meanings to elevate and endure. Co-creation of the story-in-the-making provides a framework for future events to become noticed and folded into the emerging story.

Re-authoring begins with our brief narrative ear as we listen for material that contradicts the dominant story, or lives outside the problem story. This material includes exceptions to the problem when it is not happening or less intense. It may involve identifying a unique outcome representing experiences that are different or outside the problem story. White (2011) began to substitute the term "initiative" for the terms "exception" and "unique outcome". The term initiative implies a greater sense of personal agency and intention in shaping one's life. Once identified, initiatives, exceptions and/or unique outcomes are detailed and linked together into the story-in-the-making.

Openings to possibility are heard in the gaps in the problem story. We then invite people to make sense of these events, asking questions that weave between three distinct categories of questions. The questions take us places together, so to speak, and allow for reflection, linking, and connecting events together and to broader intentions for life. We describe these categories as landscapes. Once again, geographic metaphor serves us well, invoking imaginary spaces, places, territories, or domains of experience across which we can wander and explore together, eventually arriving somewhere more preferred.

Landscape of Action

The first set of questions, referred to as "landscape of action questions", invite people to identify preferred events and the details of those events (White & Epston, 1990). These events can be located in very distant history through to the near now, providing a galaxy of experience to draw from. This involves direct inquiry about initiatives. These questions evoke the details of who, what, where, when, how, and then what.

- Tell me about a time when things are going a little better?
- How did you make that happen?
- How did you prepare yourself to make that happen?
- What did your child/partner/friend notice you doing that made a difference?
- What were the steps leading up to this? What happened just before and after?
- Where were you when this development happened?
- When did this take place?
- Who was around that supported this development?

A close examination of these questions reveals that they are presuppositional in style. The phrasing implies there *have* been times when things have been better and directs attention to those experiences. For many, to be asked about a time when things were better has them pause to research their experience as it's a question rarely asked when someone shares their concerns. I give space for their consideration and at times invite them to take a few more seconds to recall an example. I do not ask "*has* there ever been a time…" as that phrasing does not require the person to research their history and they can quickly answer "no" especially if mired in the dominance of the problem story. As we understand that there is a great deal of material outside the problem story that goes unnoticed and un-storied, presuppositional phrasing helps this to come forward.

At times, transitioning conversation from the complaint to the landscape of action requires a preamble to assist with the change in topic. This prevents the question from being too unusual and misplaced in the flow of the conversation. I may say, "I think I'm starting to get a picture of what you have been through and I'm wondering if it's okay if I ask a different kind of question that might take the conversation in different direction?" I may follow this up with sharing why I am wanting to ask a different kind of question embracing transparency. "The reason is because I imagine there are times when it hasn't always been like that, perhaps when you have refused to let this problem be the boss of you, or you were able to carry on despite it." After receiving affirmation, "Can you tell me more about those times and perhaps give me an example?" Transitions and transparency assist to accommodate people to the unique focus of the landscape of action inquiry.

"How" questions have a long history in the brief therapies for important reasons. They not only imply the person contributed to the better times but also serve to elevate the experience of personal agency. How did you do that? How did you decide to do that? How did you know to do that? All these phrasings elicit the contribution of the participant and facilitate the experience that they were able to shape their life in some way. Answers to these questions reflect the personal know-how or insider knowledge that can be further canvased and brought into proposals for action in the third phase of our encounter.

"What" questions assist to elicit further details of the preferred events. What did others notice you doing? What steps did you take leading up to this? What did you do just before or after? These are the kinds of questions that elicit the minutia of thoughts and actions that contribute to more preferred times. The details matter as they provide the context specific efforts people have engaged in that make a difference.

The "where" and "when" questions serve to further situate difference in the dimensions of time and place providing clues as to the influence of environment and timing. Last, "who" questions elicit important relationships that play a part in more preferred times. We can learn about the history of those relationships and the ways they shape the persons view of self.

As an example, a young man I met was looking to get his life back on track as he was failing school and in conflict with family. He described an event in which his friends were consuming drugs and had become out of control and ill. He noted that he hadn't taken much of the drug that day. In exploring this event, I asked, how did you manage not to get as out of control as the others? He described to me how he *pretended* to take the drugs, then passed them along to someone else. Each time they came to him, he again pretended and passed them along. When asked how he knew to do that he linked this to his "quick thinking" that helped him come up with the idea on the spot. He speculated that his family would have been proud of this initiative.

This event, within the landscape of action, provides a trace of a potential story-in-the-making related to this person's preferred future. He went on to say how he had realized how bad they look when so intoxicated and that he didn't want to be seen that way. That statement hinted at a wish for his future. I could have asked, "How would he like to be seen and known by people?" This question moves us into what White (2007) describes as the landscape of meaning.

Landscape of Meaning

The second set of questions, most commonly referred to as "landscape of meaning questions", invite people's interpretations of those preferred events (White & Epston, 1990). They invite people to reflect on the event and share the sense they make of it. Questions have people discern from their actions what they may speak to regarding concepts such as hopes for their life, wishes for things to be different, values they hold dear, intentions for life, purposes they hold, preferred identity; who they are becoming, certain qualities they represent, and skills they have developed. These questions expand the meaning related to the action/event(s) that took place.

- What do you suppose that says about the hopes you have for your relationship with…?
- What does that action say about what is important to you—what you value? (Values)
- What went into taking that step at this point in time in your life? (Skills)
- What does it say to us about who you are becoming? (Preferred identity)
- When you took this step, what does it say you were intending for your life? (Intentions)

Returning to the young man's decision to pretend to take drugs, exploring the landscape of meaning, multiple understandings became visible. The step reflected his hope for a drug free future. It made visible his intention to grow a healthier life characterized by having meaningful employment and family. It was a step towards his idea about how he would like to be seen by people closest to him. When I asked, "What does this suggest about what might be possible for you:" he responded, "A different future than a life of drugs. "

Landscape of Place

I have added a third category to Whites' map called the "landscape of place", referring to material related to descriptions of context, culture and setting. Context is ever present in narrative thinking as people live out their lives in different relational and institutional contexts such as home, work, culture and spirituality. To share in vivid story development, detailed descriptions of place and context where preferred events take place are useful. This landscape comprises questions eliciting these details, as well as sensory recall related to the events.

- Take me back to that moment. Where were you?
- What was the colour of the wallpaper?
- What was the weather like?

- What smells or sounds were you aware of?
- What were you experiencing in your body?
- What cultural teachings did you draw from that shaped your response? Who have you learned that from?
- What kinds of expectations did the world have about how to live in those days? How did you resist those gender expectations?
- What did your spiritual beliefs give to you in that moment that made such a difference?

Once again returning to our vignette, landscape of place questions assisted the young man to revisit his moment of success to recall the details of his actions. He was able to describe the nuances of his step, responding to questions such as:

- Take me back there to that moment, what time of day was this?
- Where were you?
- Were you feeling an uneasy feeling about the events about to unfold?
- Was that uneasy feeling like your warning bells going off?

Tuning into the place of his felt experience in his body was a novel understanding for him. In recall, he supposed he had listened to his *warning bells*,[1] an uneasy nervousness that alerted him to think fast. It reflected an important decision he had made in the moment for his life however this event on its own remained vulnerable to being discounted or overshadowed by many other poorer decisions.

Linking Questions

A lone event thoroughly explored, however, does not make a story. It is vulnerable to fading away or being discounted. You'll recall story structure is comprised of events *linked* together across time according to a theme. Linking actions together assists the story-in-the-making to take shape and become long lasting as opposed to a blip in time. For this reason, linking questions are used to elicit further events to explore across the landscapes and to bring into the story-line. As actions are identified, we can invite the person to link those actions to other similar actions across the timeline.

- Tell me another story about when you have done this before?
- Is that another step of self-care like you were describing earlier?
- What other times have you listened to your warning bells like that?
- Was this a new development or have you resisted the thoughts of suicide before on other occasions?

Returning one last time to the story of this young man, within our conversation, he became increasingly interested in learning that he had experienced warning

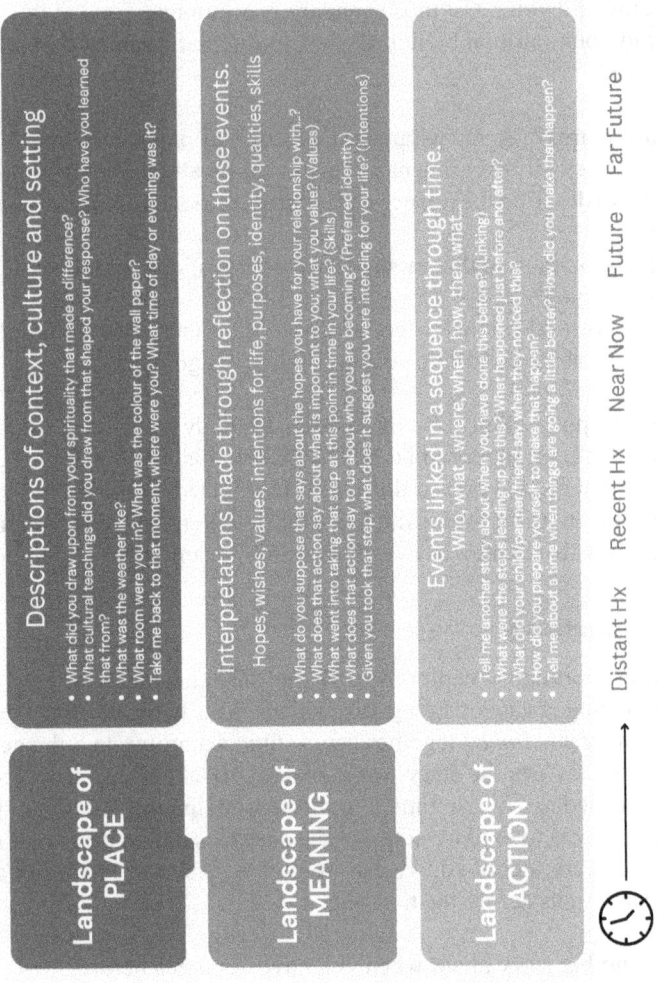

Figure 6.1 Re-authoring Stories-in-the-Making Map, adapted from White & Epston, 1990; White, M. 2007, provides a visual of the conversation landscapes. Movement through these landscapes often zig-zags throughout the domains, moving liberally throughout time–distant history, recent history, the near now, and the future.

bells and had responded to them. This was not a novel act. He started to recall other times he had resisted invitations to use drugs or limited his use. Linking these actions together and eliciting what they spoke to in terms of his intentions for his life, what they represented in terms of his skills for living, and how they represented him to those he cared about, shaped a compelling and encouraging storyline within which future decisions would fit. He came to name these actions as "Steps for My Future".

The Naming Process

Naming is a practice relevant throughout our conversation. However, it serves a specific purpose in re-authoring a story-in-the-making. It refers to inviting participants to zoom out, reflect, and give a name to the events identified comprising the emerging story-in-the-making. Throughout the middle phase, I will first invite people to ascribe a name to an identified event. I may ask questions like:

- Is that like a "step" you were taking when you did that? What was that a step towards?
- Would you call that a "skill" you were employing? What would the name of that skill be, something like "quick thinking"?
- What would you call that action you took? Was that like "self-care"?

Very often, these competencies are hardly known or visible to people. Naming them helps grow a pre-concept to a fuller concept[2] that may serve people in the future. For instance, in naming a "step of self-care" as an umbrella term, other developments perhaps not previously considered may also fit the term "self-care". It's important to note that I am not naming the development for people. I may offer suggestions; however, the name is best coming from the person themselves.

The naming practice becomes more important as part of a re-authoring conversation. As we have had participants identify unique outcomes, initiatives, or exceptions across time, we can ask if these are preferred developments and begin to seek a name reflecting the linkages of preferred developments. I often invite people to consider metaphors such as a journey, life project, chapter of life, or even steps along a path.

- Okay, so if you put all these initiatives together and were to give them a name that reflects the journey you're on, what would you call it? *The Journey Towards the Light Side of Life!*
- When you look back at these developments, what title would you give this journey you have embarked on?

- What would be a useful way to think about all these steps everyone has taken, would you call it a journey, or some sort of life project? *Our Family Peace Project!*
- Suppose we thought of these developments as a new chapter in your life, what title might you give it? *Well, the old chapter would be called the life from hell, so this chapter would be The New Beginning!*

This way of co-crafting names allows for a noticeable separation between the problem and what people want for themselves. As you see in the last bullet point, a name can be given to the problem story to contrast with the story-in-the-making. This juxtaposition helps people to experience their personal agency, understanding that they are taking previously unnoticed actions to address their circumstance.

This is highly relevant to single session work because naming the story-in-the-making creates, even while it is taking form, a framework within which to place future developments that fit. After the session, people will be more likely to notice those events, storying them within the named theme. For instance, the next time the young man experiences that uneasy feeling, he will understand it as a warning bell. Future actions to resist drugs are part of further steps for his future. Naming serves to assist the story-in-the-making to endure and continue to shape people's future meaning making. A story is much more enduring than a grouping of strategies, coping ideas, or instructions.

Re-authoring provides a map for the middle phase of the conversation. It orients us to the practice of story expansion, helping to assist people to get somewhere useful. Phase two can involve other types of conversations, such as externalizing, counter-story development, re-membering, response-based, point of reference, or hypothetical futures, to name a few. However, the re-authoring map serves as an overarching framework, linking events across time, bringing these conversations into themed stories-in-the-making.

These are often highly de-contextualized conversations typified by wonder, speculation, and negotiation of meaning. The questions within the map provide distancing, the means by which people incrementally move towards greater possibility away from the narrow and constraining meanings they arrive with. However, the task remains to begin to translate what we've talked about into doable next steps and action plans that will live on long past our talk. This requires an emphasis on the third phase of the rite of passage with a focus on endings.

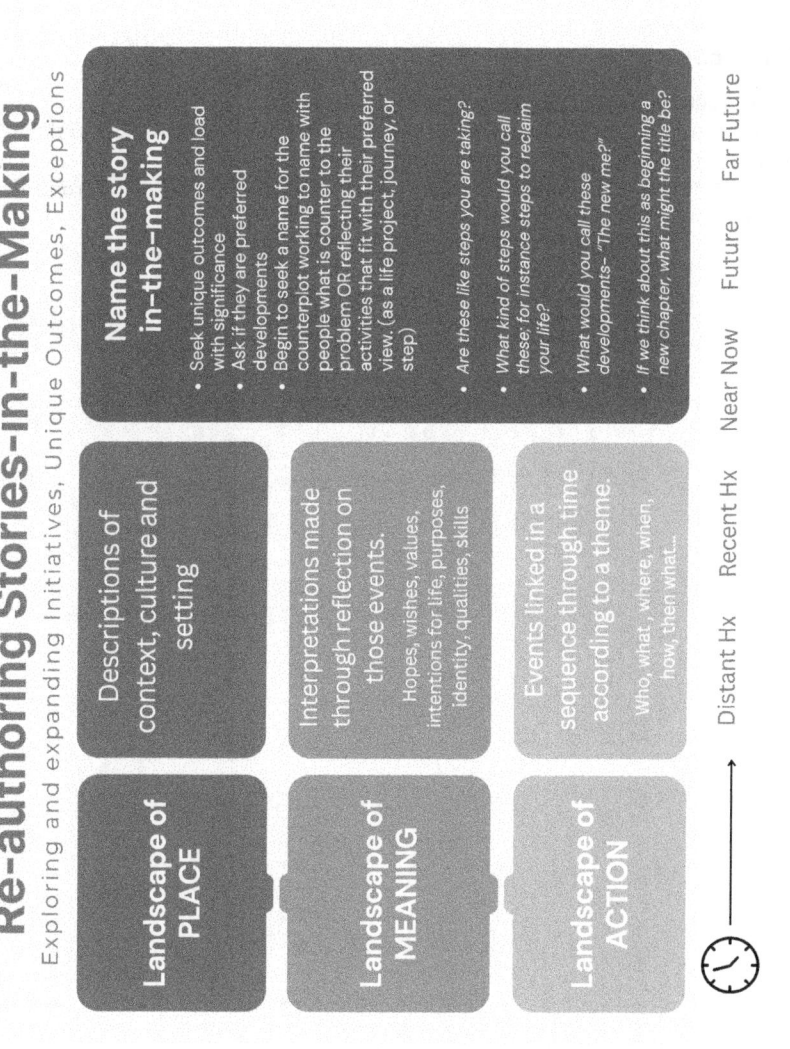

Re-authoring Stories-in-the-Making

Exploring and expanding Initiatives, Unique Outcomes, Exceptions

Name the story in-the-making

- Seek unique outcomes and load with significance
- Ask if they are preferred developments
- Begin to seek a name for the counterplot working to name with people what is counter to the problem OR reflecting their activities that fit with their preferred view. (as a life project, journey, or step)

- *Are these like steps you are taking?*
- *What kind of steps would you call these; for instance steps to reclaim your life?*
- *What would you call these developments–"The new me?"*
- *If we think about this as beginning a new chapter, what might the title be?*

Landscape of PLACE

Descriptions of context, culture and setting

Landscape of MEANING

Interpretations made through reflection on those events.

Hopes, wishes, values, intentions for life, purposes, identity, qualities, skills

Landscape of ACTION

Events linked in a sequence through time according to a theme.

Who, what , where, when, how, then what...

Distant Hx   Recent Hx   Near Now   Future   Far Future

Figure 6.2 Re-authoring Stories-in-the-Making Map, adapted from White & Epston, 1990; White, M. 2007, with emphasis on naming practice to assist the story-in-the-making to endure.

Notes

1 This is an example of languaging into existence the concept of 'warning bells' through the action of meaning making.
2 See Chapter 17 for ideas related to the development of concepts in single session therapy.

References

White, M. (2007). *Maps of narrative practice*. New York: W.W. Norton.
White, M. (2011). *Narrative practice: Continuing the conversations*. New York: W.W. Norton.
White, M. & Epston, D. (1990). *Narrative means to therapeutic ends*. New York: W.W. Norton.

Chapter 7

Phase Three: Conversation Endurance

As the opening phase is concerned with coming together, embarking on a journey and separating from the old ways of the outside world, the closing phase is about arriving at a more preferred destination. In this chapter, we turn our attention to the third phase of the process and specifically ways to assist the conversation to endure long past the face-to-face contact.

Through the metaphor of the rites of passage the third phase of reincorporation highlights a time of arrival at a new destination or status. People re-enter everyday life not as who they were but with new possibilities if not expectations for how to be. This arrival is often publicly marked through celebration and public participation.

Conversation endurance is a concept I have been exploring for many years. I think back to conversations in my life that have had lasting effects or stayed with me assisting my life journey. Teasing out the ingredients of those conversations, I am drawn to how context specific they were to my life. I could relate to what was being said and fit it into my life. They involved a mood of speculation with a theme of "what if" or a sense of "becoming". It is this mood of relevance and possibility we seek to conjure in the third phase of single session therapy.

As guidance for this project, I have concerned myself with the following questions:

- How do we assist stories-in-the-making to live on, endure, and resist being overshadowed by problem stories after a single session?
- How can we have a conversation that forms a setting for events or next steps fitting with developing preferred story lines to take place and be noticed?
- How can we inoculate an emerging preferred story against assimilation into problematic plot lines?

These spawn from the idea that all conversations are at risk of fading. Further, problem stories can be difficult to dislodge as they are often widely known, sometimes have been around for a long time, or are well supported by the context of people's lives. Given this, this chapter will share the micro-practices

DOI: 10.4324/9781003431688-8

involved in shoring up stories-in-the-making that last and influence people's outside world.

Within many traditions of therapeutic practice, it is not uncommon for the therapist to prescribe a task, intervention, or homework that the therapy participants are to complete between sessions and then report back on to the therapist. In a single session encounter, the one contact we have could be the one and only contact with that family. Given this arrangement, follow-up in relation to task completion or usefulness of the task is not likely. Further, in the process of task prescription, the therapist typically takes the lead role in determining which task(s) would fit and then offers their ideas. Efforts to convince and justify to participants the usefulness of the task and the importance of their commitment to the task can accompany this.

Centering the therapists' ideas in this way can prove hazardous in single session therapy. The participants may receive meta-messages that the therapist is viewing them as incapable of coming up with their own ideas or perhaps that their own ideas are not useful. The meta-message of incapability may erode their sense of personal agency. Second, suppose the participants commit to the task and it fails them. There is a risk that they story this experience as personal failure. Last, these assigned tasks that centre the therapists' ideas risk being contextually and culturally incongruent with the life of the participants. They lack the specificity that is part of a person's life and culture. This contextual and cultural gap between prescribed tasks and real life works against success and the usefulness of any sort of next step. Worst case, they can be unsafe for people to execute.

For these reasons, I resist prescribing tasks or homework and have sought other ways to extend the influence of the conversation. Embracing a brief narrative perspective, the project is to get on to more preferred stories that people can live. The rest of this chapter will outline this process and its rationale. We will look at the concepts of session retellings, reflecting surface, receiving context and explore a map of inquiry that incorporates these concepts making for enduring conversation.

Session Re-Telling

Watching Michael's work with families, it was clear he used variations of "summary" at certain points in the conversation. Nearing the end of session, he would share back much of what he heard, drawing from his notes and the specific words and phrases spoken. This makes some sense as he premised his work on tellings and re-tellings of stories to generate meaning-making skills. Jim Duvall at Brief Training Centres International™ had been refining this practice of a specific kind of summary over many years formally highlighting the use of "session summaries" in narrative conversations to transition into ending conversations (Duvall & Béres, 2011). They introduced the idea of these summaries being more extensive, looking back over the entire session. What was understood and written down is reviewed for accuracy and the emerging alternate story held up for reflection.

Bringing these ideas into brief narrative conversations, I have continued to refine the practice and call them "session re-tellings". A session re-telling is similarly positioned to what Duvall and Béres suggest as a segue to the ending of the conversation. It is a storied recount of what has been shared and how it fits into emerging storylines discussed in the session. This differs from summarizing, in which one may read back a sort of bullet list of what was discussed. Re-tellings involve plot and character development. In this sharing, I take license to dramatize the re-telling to provide an interesting and energizing narrative that's meaningful and unfolding. The dramatization does not mean I take authorship of the developing story. I stay as close as possible to what we have talked about using the persons' own words or our agreed upon language. I check in throughout the re-telling with them to be sure I am re-telling with some accuracy.

Dramatization may involve emphasizing specific words, inserting pauses for emphasis and using inflection to have story elements stand out. It may involve foregrounding the protagonist/antagonist struggle, juxtaposing their intentions, and highlighting the ways the protagonist has turned the tide or emerged from the oppression of the protagonist (externalized Problem). I may re-tell what I heard pitting the story-in-the-making up against the problem saturated dominant narrative to further elicit one's preferences.

There is a structure to these re-tellings. First, I elicit permission to share back what has stood out for me to this point in our time together to provide a segue into phase three.

I'm just aware of the time. Would it be okay if I share back what I've heard so far and then perhaps we can look at some next steps?

I'm wondering if this would be a good time for me to share some of the highlights of our conversation and please correct me if I've misunderstood and then we can discuss ideas to try out when you leave here today if you think that would be useful?

With permission granted, I begin by noting what my understanding was about why the participant or family came in and the agreed upon purpose of our time together. I will share why this is important momentarily.

So, when you came today, you noted you wanted to talk most about your experience of depression...

I then highlight standout parts of the conversation, including meaningful exceptions or initiatives, important ideas, useful metaphors, significant moments, and also the potential implications of such ideas. This could involve noting a climax, turning point, act of resistance, or critical juncture that arose. It may foreground people's actions, responses, and the emerging storyline. It may bring the problem story and the story-in-the-making into collision and juxtaposition, spotlighting people's preference for the story-in-the-making. It may revisit a future focus.

It is at that point in which I will invite people to "thematicize" through ascribing a title or name to the emerging plot just prior to eliciting the next steps if one has not yet already emerged.

> So, looking back on these developments, if you could give this emerging pro-ject a name, what might you call it?

> This seems like you are beginning to write a very different chapter in coming here today. If you were to give it a name, what might you title it?

We often understand these plots as life projects, quests, experiments, journeys of some sort. As noted previously, naming serves to hold up a future theme in which new information can be situated. This title may offer a shift in attitude towards the problem or re-define how things are going to be different living with the problem.

The session re-telling is brief, much like a highlight reel and serves several important roles. At this juncture in the conversation, it allows for what Bateson (1972) termed the perception of difference. He notes that all receipt of informa-tion draws upon the receipt of "news of difference". If that recounted difference is too slight, it will not be perceived. If it is too wide, it may be discounted. We want to represent a difference in the re-telling that is easily perceived.

As mentioned, to achieve this I share back the reason they come in for the session and contrast it to where we have arrived, given our recent conversation. Difference between when one came in (known and familiar) and what they are now coming to understand (possible to know) fits within the metaphor of the single session being "a step" on the journey and offers a perceptible difference.

Further, the perception of difference is a hope friendly experience. By that I mean for therapy participants it invites the sense that they are not where they were when they came in. Within this one conversation, they have movement. They may experience this as a sense of personal agency (I can do something) and recall options (I know what to do) for the next step. Perception of difference is the antidote to hopelessness.

Reflecting Surface: The Springboard for Discerning Next Steps

I likened using a session re-telling in this way to when people look into a mirror. In seeing our reflection, we find ourselves in a position to look at our appearance and decide about altering it, such as combing our hair. We engage in deciding about what to do, if anything. Without the mirror, it would be difficult to know what needs altering and what should be left alone. In discerning and deciding, we are exercising our personal agency; the ability to direct our lives. With the aid of the mirror, we achieve a different vantage point from which to view ourselves.

Similarly, in observing a river, one has a different experience and view when standing at the top of a cliff, on the shoreline, or from within the river itself. From different vantage points, it affords us different perspectives from which to decide what to do next. A session re-telling serves as a reflecting surface (White 2007) and allows people to be an audience to the movie of their life. It's the different vantage point that favours reflexivity. "This reflexivity is a capacity to achieve distance in relation to the immediacy of life" Michael White (2004, p. 91).

Rennie (1992), links client's reflexivity to playing a role in therapeutic change. He refers to the reflexive moment as a "safety zone" in which a course of action is contemplated, a decision about how to proceed reached and then turned into action. He notes further, "It is in the reflexivity that the individual has choices, and hence the possibility of control over change" (p. 227–228). In this reflexive place, people can consider and adopt perspectives that have been explored in our conversation and that differ from their subjective standpoints. It is an ability to review the events of our lives from other vantage points. "It is in the reflexive moment that intentions are formed… seeking follow-through" (p. 227). In these moments, we contemplate a course of action.

Similarly, White (2004) speaks of the reflexive position as providing some distance from the immediacy of experience. It provides a reflecting surface (White, 2007) to view, giving an opportunity for them to reflect upon their words, meanings, and life events, as well as what the therapist has heard. Reflexivity in therapy is a moment in which the participant is freed from a respondent position to assume a reflexive stance as audience that helps them consider the conversation and process. Therefore, it is in sharing back the account of the session that the therapist is holding the concepts up and apart from the participant as a reflecting surface or mirror to view and examine. This provides opportunity for the participant to distance from previously held concepts, experience-near effects of the story told, assisting them to ponder and propose potential next steps they hadn't previously considered.

Participants stand outside their own shoes and re-engage with their past in a different light. A menu of options may emerge which participants can take up in their lives through consideration, choice, and decision to act. The therapist can then archive these proposals for action/next steps, gathering them into a plan that is a fit and is relevant to the participant(s). However, even though ideas may emerge about next steps, the translation into practice in the real world is desired. When asked, people will come up with proposals for action that are relevant to them. However, the context within which these next steps take place may need to be shifted.

Receiving Context

Life presents a panorama of meaning and interpretation of events from which people form and tell the stories of their lives. However, the stories that we hold about life can constrain and limit possibility. David Epston, in interpreting the work of Gregory Bateson, notes, "… he proposed that the understanding we have of, or the meaning we ascribe to any event is determined and restrained by the receiving context for the event, that is by the network of premises and presuppositions that constitute our map of the world… the interpretation of any event was determined by how it fit with known patterns of events…" (White & Epston, 1990, p.2). The concept of "receiving context" has taken on great relevance in our therapeutic practice and especially in single session practice.

In consideration of Bateson's ideas, it is the stories that people hold that provide the receiving context for experience. The receiving context is composed of the "premises and presuppositions we have that contribute to our worldview" (p. 2). It refers to the emerging future frame in which concepts find acceptance. The effect of the receiving context is to constrain what we conceive of as possible and what we pay attention to or notice.

You have likely had the experience of an altered receiving context in your life. For instance, if you have been thinking about buying a new car and were interested in a particular brand of vehicle, say a Caravan, when you are out in the community it is likely you notice many more Caravans than you had before becoming interested in buying one. You start to see them driving by you, in commercials, or may even notice your neighbour has one. That is the effect of receiving context. In narrowing your search to Caravans, you have developed a receiving context much friendlier to Caravan sightings. This process is similar for therapy participants.

Suppose a person entered therapy with a very dominant problem-saturated story of being a failure in their profession. This problem story of failure would serve as a receiving context for other experiences that fit with the frame or theme of failure and that confirmed the failure storyline. The dominant story serves as a filter of meaning; filtering those events out of the panorama of life that fit with the most dominant known and familiar story.

Duvall and Béres (2011) have brought discussion specific to addressing the receiving contexts of people's emerging stories into the therapeutic conversation. In a single session encounter, receiving context becomes very central to the development of next steps or plans for action. Given that the first contact is likely the last contact, it is important to address and counter receiving contexts that support dominant problem-saturated stories. The development of the story-in-the-making in a single session remains highly vulnerable to old problem saturated receiving contexts. We can engage in a conversation that develops a receiving context that is more supportive of the emerging preferred story rather than the old problem story. Discussion of the receiving context serves to set the stage for noticing and incorporation of future initiatives into the story-in-the-making.

Turning again to Michael Whites' live demonstrations, over the years I had noticed that nearing the end of these single session consultations, he would ask the participant if it would be useful for them to have the strategies or ideas that they had co-developed with them when they needed them the most. Engaging them in speculation, he would go on to ask about what difference it would make to them if they had those ideas in their time of need? These questions intrigued me, and I speculated about how they were useful to people. Would these lines of inquiry assist people to leave with more options to address their problem? Did it also contribute to the person's sense that they could do something soon to address their concern? I realized these questions, although quite speculative, were altering the person's future frame of reference, their receiving context. Narratives with themes of helplessness, hopelessness, and futility had shifted to alternative narratives of agency, hope, and possibility. Yet the question remained, how could these alternative stories endure past the single session conversation?

Combining these ideas, the following represents a Conversation Endurance Map of progressive questions that follow the session re-telling to facilitate the co-development of actions, to alter receiving context, and to address constraints to change. See Figure 7.1.

Discern Next Steps

Following the session retelling we are ready to invite people to come up with what I refer to as *next steps* to be taken following the session. This involves asking specific questions, inviting people to come up with their own ideas about what to try out, keep doing, or to take away with them from the conversations. I invite them to translate their know-how into plans of actions.

- What thoughts do you have about steps that might follow this conversation?
- Given what we have talked about, what ideas are coming to mind about a next step you can take when you leave here today?
- Given our conversation, what will you practice when you leave here that will start the ball rolling?
- What might be possible to do that would be more in harmony with what you value, what you are learning that's really important to you?
- What steps might you take to address this situation?

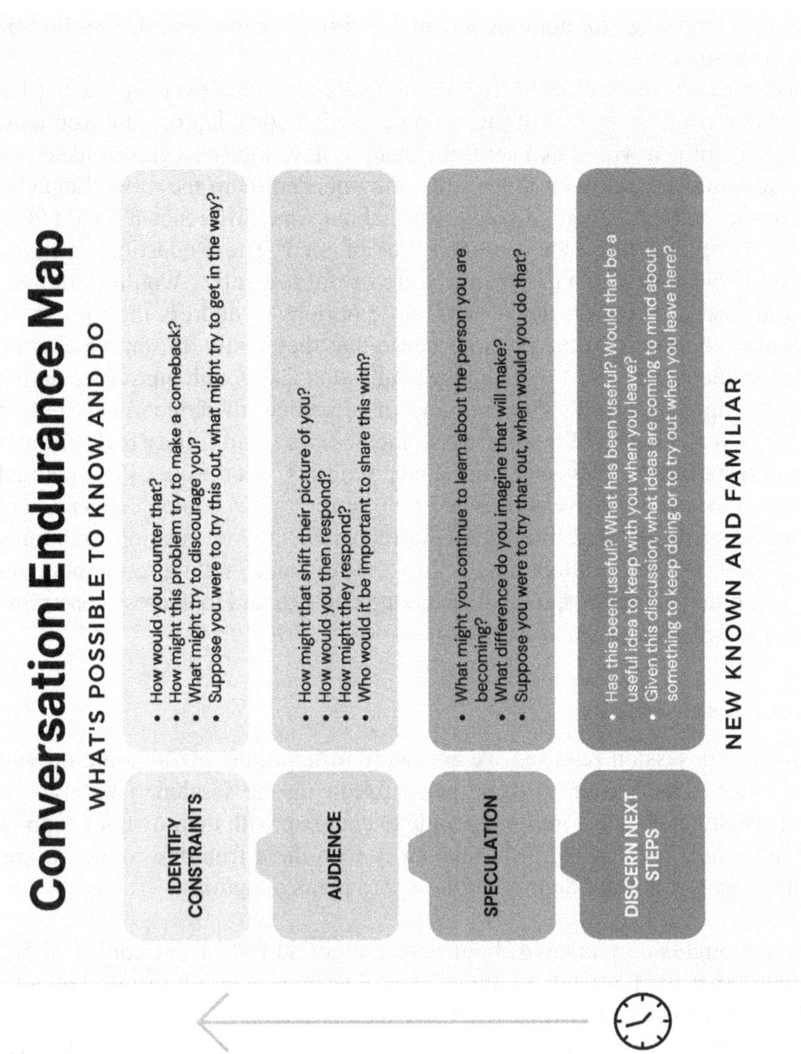

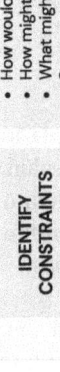

Conversation Endurance Map

WHAT'S POSSIBLE TO KNOW AND DO

IDENTIFY CONSTRAINTS
- How would you counter that?
- How might this problem try to make a comeback?
- What might try to discourage you?
- Suppose you were to try this out, what might try to get in the way?

AUDIENCE
- How might that shift their picture of you?
- How would you then respond?
- How might they respond?
- Who would it be important to share this with?

SPECULATION
- What might you continue to learn about the person you are becoming?
- What difference do you imagine that will make?
- Suppose you were to try that out, when would you do that?

DISCERN NEXT STEPS
- Has this been useful? What has been useful? Would that be a useful idea to keep with you when you leave?
- Given this discussion, what ideas are coming to mind about something to keep doing or to try out when you leave here?

NEW KNOWN AND FAMILIAR

Figure 7.1 Phase three conversation endurance map.

- What's the next step on the journey when you leave here?
- What would be the first step in making that happen?

Sometimes it is also a matter of continuing to do what has been useful to date.

- What is your idea about what to keep doing when you leave here today?
- Given our conversation, what ideas are coming to mind to try out or to keep doing that has already been making a difference to you?

Speculation to Contextualize

The next level of questions serves to invite people to contextualize the next steps into their everyday living and relationships. I ask questions that elicit speculated details of the effects of implementing their ideas, the initiatives, into the everyday and beyond. This can move through the timeline into the near and distant future. Freedman and Combs (2002) have also highlighted these questions to "extend the story into the future" (p.35). More recent explorations have linked this line of questioning to "futures discourse" to foster anticipatory action learning (Milojević, 2014). Through this speculation, I am also assisting the receiving context to shift to be more friendly to the incorporation of future preferred developments.

- What difference will that make to try out these ideas when you leave here?
- How long do you suppose you'll need to practice that?
- How will it affect what you do when you leave today?
- What small effects will this have on your life?
- How will these effects be celebrated?
- At what time do you predict you'll make this happen?
- What will you be wearing?
- What will you say as you do that?
- How will you use this conversation summary?
- Where will you keep it?
- When will you read it?
- What difference will it make to you having these ideas somewhere where you can read them and review them?

These speculations can be of a wild and exaggerated nature to facilitate possibility. This further speaks to inquiring about the particularities for the actions people become inspired to take. I am seeking to engage their imagination.

Audience

"The scope of these alternative stories can be further extended through introducing questions that invite persons to identify and recruit an audience to the performance of new meanings in their life" (White & Epston, 1990, p. 41). I appreciate how Duvall and Béres (2011) talk about inquiring about audience as "a receiving context that is inhabited by others who validate and support the efforts of people to perform their new story makes them far less vulnerable to the influence of the old problem story" (p.84). This inquiry involves specific questions about the other characters mentioned in the session and their contribution to a person's life when they leave. This is a re-contextualization of the conversation into the social realm of people's lives and sets the stage for the noticing of their preferred responses.

- Who would be the first to notice your efforts? How might they respond?
- Who will it be meaningful to share this conversation with?
- Who will it be important to have read this document?
- Who may notice what about you that they hadn't before?
- How will their image of you shift when they hear about this conversation?
- How might they respond?
- Suppose they respond as expected, what would that be like for you and how might you respond next?

Addressing Constraints

Dominant narratives can be very hard to shift, and the circumstances of life may play out to keep people mired in the old ways of being. To predict and counter these circumstances, I invite people to speculate and discuss potential constraints to the story-in-the-making. As we identify constraints, counter actions can be planned as needed. This is often a place in which we discuss safety, as sometimes safety can become compromised if people plan to make changes in their lives.

- What constraints may make themselves known trying to keep the problem in your life?
- How might the problem try to maintain its hold on you?
- How would you counter its strategies?
- What may try to get in the way of your practice?
- What might happen that tries to take you backwards or off-track?
- How will you handle that hurdle, pothole, back step?

This element of the discussion serves to render the influence of problems more visible and draws forth the creativity and preparedness of participants for the struggle that can accompany people trying to bring their lives in accordance with their preferences.

Navigating through the Conversation Endurance Map sets the stage for practice in the real world following the single session. I talk about experimenting or trying out what we have discussed and seeing how it goes. We are implying that there is work to be done and more can happen outside the single session. We are setting the scene for these conversations to ripple out into everyday life, like a rain drop creating ripples in a puddle.

I also invite the participant(s) to establish a period of time for practice before considering further services. Too often I have seen therapists co-develop a doable, contextualized action plan with someone only to add information to call for a referral to further services as another step. To me, this is like suggesting the single session conversation and the next steps we just spent time co-crafting are not going to be useful.

We cannot know ahead of time the influence of these conversations. For this reason, it's important to establish a period of practice prior to consideration of more services.

How long do you suppose you'll have to practice this before making a decision about future services?

How often do you think you'll have to practice this before it starts to make a difference or has it already started to make a difference?

I may also invite people to 'see how it goes' and then return to the walk-in as sometimes plans need some adjusting or fine-tuning along the way. I am assuming our conversation will be enough, will ripple and reverberate in their real life.

This chapter completes the three phases of a single session encounter. It has outlined the process to assist people to come up with next steps to address their concern following a single session. In the third phase, we are inviting people to translate the conversation into action plans or contextualized next steps that assist the conversation to endure and the story-in-the-making to grow. It is important that there is some sense of certainty on the person's behalf that they can accomplish the ideas they set out to achieve. Ideas that are not achievable risk setting the scene for the experience of personal failure. Achievable next steps maintain the momentum of the performance of the emerging preferred story.

References

Bateson, G. (1972). *Steps to an ecology of mind.* New York: Chandler.

Duvall, J. & Béres, L. (2011). *Innovations in narrative therapy: Connecting practice, training, and research.* New York: W. W. Norton.

Freedman, J. & Combs, G. (2002). *Narrative therapy with couples… and a whole lot more! A collection of papers, essays and exercises.* Adelaide, Dulwich Centre Publications.

Milojević, I. (2014). Creating alternative selves: The use of futures discourse in narrative therapy. *Journal of Futures Studies*, March *18*(3), 27–40.

Rennie, D. L. (1992). Qualitative analysis of the client's experience: The unfolding of reflexivity. In S. G. Toukmanian & D. L. Rennie (Eds.), *Psychotherapy process research: Pragmatic and narrative approaches* (pp. 211–234). Newbury Park, CA: Sage Publications.

White, M. (2004). Working with people who are suffering the consequences of multiple trauma: A narrative perspective. *International Journal of Narrative Therapy and Community Work*, (1), 45–76. Reprinted in D. Denborough, (Ed.). (2006). *Trauma: Narrative responses to traumatic experience* (pp. 25–85). Adelaide, Australia: Dulwich Centre Publications.

White, M. (2007). *Maps of narrative practice*. W.W. Norton, New York.

White, M. & Epston, D. (1990). *Narrative means to therapeutic ends*. New York: W.W. Norton.

Chapter 8

Co-Crafting Take-Away Documents

Therapeutic tradition and often agency policies require a "case note" or recording, archiving various aspects of therapeutic discussion. Typically, that task occurs post session with a reliance on the professional to recall and record the required information. This act is often done in private without the input of the participant, free of their feedback and review. In such a process, there is a risk of privileging the professional's voice and understandings over the participants. This is opportunity lost, as those archives can play an important part in contributing to the therapeutic process.

The exploration and use of therapeutic documents in working with people and families has a long history in narrative practice (White & Epston, 1990; White 1995, 2000; Freedman and Coombs, 1996; Freeman, Epston and Lobovits, 1997). I have been experimenting with crafting therapeutic documents during single session conversations for some time now. The co-creation of what I call "take-away documents" in SST has become a very important, creative, and fun part of the process.

I refer to these documents as take-away documents as we craft them within the single session with the intention of them going with the person consulting to us and perhaps finding a wider circulation with a fitting audience. The work of Michael White, David Epston (White & Epston, 1990; White, 1995), who introduced co-crafting therapeutic documents as part of narrative therapy, fully inspired this practice. In the time-constrained context of single session therapy, their usefulness finds even greater importance. These documents are co-crafted, that is, crafted together with participant (s) during the conversation as you go. The production of documents within the single session serves many practical and ethical purposes. Before we come to that, let's look more closely at the practice of collaborative documentation.

Collaborative Documentation

Common practice in brief narrative therapy is to take notes as we talk (Epston & White, 1990; Freedman & Combs, 2002; Young, Dick, Herring & Lee, 2008).

DOI: 10.4324/9781003431688-9

These notes are not kept private though or contain only the therapists' ideas. The notes are co-developed and co-crafted, along with the participant within the session. This is a form of collaborative concurrent documentation as we engage the participants in identifying not only what should be included in the document but also how to phrase what is recorded. This involves intentional periodic pauses to check in to ask for participants' advice.

- Okay, should we get that down on this document?
- Would that be an important idea to get on this document to keep with you when you leave?
- I have this space in the conversation summary to describe the problem. How should I phrase what you have been sharing?
- How did you say that again? I just want to be sure to get it down correctly.

Other times, I will begin a sentence out loud and then gesture to the participant to complete it. This is an invitation to take up authorship and contribute, in their own words, information that would be useful to keep with them after the session. Collaborating in this way guards against the risk of foregrounding our own voice, interpretations, and understandings over participants. It helps to ensure the document remains clear and relevant to the participant.

While collaborative documentation is a skill that may require practice, it serves many purposes. Not only is it an efficient use of time, the process reflects our view that participants are knowledgeable and we are partners on this journey. Writing down their phrases and words helps people to see themselves in these documents, avoiding jargon that may be distancing. The therapist does not have to rely on recall post session as paperwork requirements are completed by the end of the session. The document is uploaded into the agency's data base.

Benefits of Co-Crafting Take-Away Documents

In co-crafting the document, we are creating a context favourable to the experience of personal agency. In the moment of co-authorship, participants experience doing something about the problem. They are taking action and intervening in their life. That experience of personal agency fosters a sense of hope and possibility.

Documents also archive peoples' own knowledge as opposed to only professional knowledge. The recorded know-how is very nuanced. It reflects what people learned, the skills and ideas they draw upon each day. As a brief narrative therapist, it's my responsibility to invite people to mentor me in their know-how and to collect it up with them so it may be put to use. Collecting that know-how in a take-away document keeps it in the foreground so it's more accessible when needed. By keeping their ideas and skills present in this concrete way, it's less likely to be forgotten or overshadowed by the problem as people return to the context of their lives. People engage in self consultation as they can consult their own knowledgeableness (White, 1995).

White (2000, p. 6) highlights how documents can "contribute significantly to the visibility, substantiation, and endurance of the sparkling events that are identified in narrative conversations". Take-away documents highlight sparkling moments, initiatives, and exceptions that can be drawn together into stories-in-the-making. They elevate a developing counter-story out of the panorama of lived experience and problem-dominant accounts of life. As these documents return home with people, they extend the range of influence of the conversation beyond the face-to-face contact. They provide a receiving context for new information and ideas congruent with their focus. That creates a favourable context for the story-in-the-making to grow.

When take-away documents are shared, they help to circulate the know-how or emerging story to a meaningful audience. Audience can be invited to respond and play a greater part in assisting with the project, whatever it might be. Furthermore, when audience includes people who are experiencing similar circumstances, the documents provide useful ideas and let them know they are not alone in their experiences.

Very often, people offer a copy of their document to display in our waiting room so other families arriving at the clinic can access them. This practice places the participant in the position of consultant[1] (Epston & White, 1990; Epston, White & 'Ben', 1995) and can assist them to know they also are not alone in their concern but part of a community who may be experiencing similar struggles. To learn they may help others is often a welcomed idea.

Documenting Practices

As noted in Chapter 5, at the outset of our meeting, we ask permission to take notes and highlight that we will do our best to record their words, not ours. I note that at the conclusion of our time, they have the option to take a copy of the note with them, which we call a conversation summary. This ensures they will have a copy of what will be kept in the file. This is part of structuring safety and being transparent about what I am recording. Should they not want me to take notes as we go, I will respect that, however, it is rare for someone to decline. With permission granted, I strive to have my notes reflect people's own words and phrases or the agreed-upon language we share in.

Conversation Summaries

The Conversation Summary (CS) is the primary collaborative concurrent document I use to archive the session. Once completed, the CS serves as the record for the session and the participant is offered a copy to take with them to consult afterwards. There is no further documentation following the session, so this is an efficient practice.

The form is divided into four quadrants with headings (Korman, 2005). These sections include the top right quadrant titled "Concern" with a line for recording "Hopes for today". The top left quadrant is titled "Background". The lower left is titled "Initiatives" while the last quadrant, the lower right, is called "Next steps". I don't record everything said within the session. The idea is to archive the agreed upon key points, phrases, statements, storylines, and wonderings, that are meaningful to the process and identified as useful to the participant.

Originally, I began using the quadrant format as a training tool. It provided a useful visual aid for the practitioner as the conversation unfolded. For instance, if just the Concern quadrant was filling up, it is a cue to ask some different questions to get on to initiatives, exceptions and difference. A quadrant for Next Steps reminds the practitioner to use the re-telling to springboard into the co-development of ideas to practice in the real world. Participants appreciated the simple and clear flow of the document, so the CS has remained as our standard document. Again, in my pre-amble I have asked permission to take notes and shared that my common practice is to provide the participant with a copy of the document at the end of our time together. Let's consider each quadrant more closely.

Hopes for Today

On the line titled "Hopes for today...", I will highlight what was identified as most important to talk about given the time we have together. Noting this keeps the purpose or focus present throughout the conversation. This is important because if we stray too far from what the participant came to address, we risk eroding therapeutic alliance and usefulness of the conversation. Keeping the focus present on the conversation summary can remind us about what the participants want to talk about most. This helps therapist resist the many pulls that invite them to pursue their own agendas, interests, and wishes in conversation.

Concern

Within the "Concern" quadrant, I note the participants' description of the problem. This can include who, what, where, when, as well as the effects of the problem. For instance, I may write, "Sadness tries to get in the way of Joey doing the things he wants to do like having fun, being with friends, and liking himself". As the conversation unfolds, I may even have the opportunity to archive the co-developed name for the problem if we've begun an externalizing conversation. I am trying to archive enough about the problem so participants experience being heard and that we have honoured what they have been through. I am careful not to over detail the problem to where problem talk takes up all the airtime or is experienced as demoralizing.

Background

Under this heading I will record elements of the story that are especially meaningful and contribute to story expansion. This may include particular skills of living, interests, hobbies, threads of cherished stories, values, hopes, and/or wishes for things to be different. Very often, what is noted in this section provides a foundation for addressing concerns and highlights what people have to put up against the problems in their life. Relevant Inquiry focuses on meeting people through stories of competence, asks about specific values or beliefs they hold that guide their life, and significant relationships and cultural or spiritual influences.

Initiatives

Within this quadrant, I note what works even a little. This can include what's worked recently or in the past, including identified meaningful initiatives, exceptions, unique outcomes; those moments when the problem had less influence or was not around. It may include counter steps people have taken in the face of the problem, such as counter thoughts, feelings, and actions, as well as the steps leading to those developments. Material in this section often provides elements that can be brought into counter-story themes and informs next steps. Having "what works even a little bit" noted and available to them when they leave, can be useful to people as they can consult this information should the influence of the problem return. It can assist them to maintain hope as they are reminded of their past successes and options available to them.

Next Steps

The last quadrant notes the co-created plan or next steps the person will leave with and begin to employ. These steps can include ideas to keep with them after the session, or specific actions to experiment with to bring their life more in harmony with their preferences for living. This quadrant is informed by the conversation endurance map outlined in Chapter 7. See Appendix 3c for corresponding questions for each quadrant.

The second page of the document includes space for identifying information, recording a co-developed safety plan if that took place, as well as a blank space for creating a social genogram, if needed. It can be used to note a specific list or drawing that proved useful during the conversation.

To remain aware about risk/safety concerns, there are two check boxes on the document. One we check if no concerns were noted. The second we check if concerns were present. Underneath we note the agreed upon steps discussed to shore up safety. Keeping risk/safety present in this way ensures we do our diligence and records for the file what was done. At times, I may jump to co-craft a specific safety plan on a separate document that accompanies the CS.

Again, once completed, the document is photocopied and offered to the participants to take home for future review. The conversation summary serves as the required recording of the session many agencies call for. In this practice, participants receive an exact copy of the information kept in their file at the agency. They can circulate the document should they wish. If our translation from the spoken to the written is not as accurate as it should be, participants can seek edits.

Often, I will jump off of the conversation summary to craft one of many tailored documents to highlight specific information. I have explored several brief narrative means to develop take-away documents with the children and youth I see at the walk-in clinic. Aside from conversation summaries, I look forward to many ways to jump into creative documentation. The children inspire and often direct these jump offs in mid conversation. Whether it involves rendering visible an externalized critter, creature, or varmint that needs some training in their life, or an adventure storybook consisting of drawings of their talking tears, these moments offer opportunity to archive young people's knowledge to be revisited, shared, and appreciated.

I first preference the possible creation of a document in a preamble, noting perhaps it would be useful to craft a document collecting up the youth/families/adult's know-how. For transparency, I share my thoughts about why I am suggesting this, noting a document could be consulted after our conversation or perhaps be shared with family members or help other people who might benefit from reading it.

> I'm wondering if it would be okay if we craft a document to highlight what you were just talking about. The reason I suggest this is that I wonder if it will help keep these ideas present for you when you need them. Perhaps it could also help other who are experiencing difficulties of their own. Would it be okay if we craft together a document?

Once we reach agreement, the process is collaborative, one of co-creation in which I may take the lead, offering a phrase or partial sentence or pictorial idea, but then gesture to my conversational partner to continue on to add their ideas and images. We weave back and forth as I provide structure and guidance, often fitting with particular maps of narrative therapy. They provide the content specific to their lives. Periodically, I summarize back allowing for editing and revising as we go.

When the document is finished, I ask if they would like to take a copy with them. It's important to ask, as in some contexts it may not be safe or private enough to store a take-away document depending on its content. I also ask if they would be interested in having their document shared with other people who may face similar circumstances and who may benefit from their ideas.

I've witnessed many moments in which these documents inspire others and assure people they are not alone in experiencing distress, but are part of a collective whose ideas, when drawn upon, can shoulder each other up. Copies of take-away documents such as poems or handbooks about the problem remain in our waiting room for people to browse or consult when they arrive at the walk-in clinic. Many times, I will direct people to specific documents or invite them to add their contributions to a growing document, such as The Big Book of Taming & Training Worry Critters, Creatures, and Varmints.

Different Kinds of Take-Away Documents

Besides the conversation summary, many kinds of take-away documents can be co-authored within a single session, as we are only limited by our imagination. Some documents I often turn to include:

Lists

The practice of listing provides a very brief and useful take away document, especially for young children. I take the opportunity to list counter thoughts and/or counter talk young people employ in the face of problems. That material can be contrasted with the Problem, bringing them into juxtaposition providing an opportunity to examine their relevance.

Other times, a list may serve as a means to collect up the traces of know-how that could be put to more agentive use. Many young people come to discount or forget what they've done that has made a difference in the past. Listing this knowledge as we hear it brings it together and makes it visible. It is often the material that informs plans and next steps.

In this practice, we jointly identify and name things worth listing. Freeman and Coombs (2002 p. 167–182) speak to the many benefits of the co-development of lists with people. Among these benefits, I appreciate that lists can be continually revisited and added to. Given this, I will leave space for prospective discoveries that can be added once the participant returns home. This practice sends the meta-message that there is more to come.

This sample list brings into juxtaposition a female teenaged youth's experience of the "push for perfection" with her own self-named "wise women" ideas about life, her sense of worth and relationships. We juxtaposed what the externalized problem of Perfection wants her to think and believe with counter thoughts

Table 8.1

When My 'Wise Women' Speaks	When 'Perfection' Speaks
My kind and caring side	*Never good enough/Judgement/Worry side*
• I value kindness and deserve it too! • People want to spend time with me because I'm nice and fun! • I'm not here to impress anyone! • I'm good enough just the way I am! • Friendships are important to me. • I'm fine the way I am!	• You get cheated on because you're not good enough. • You're not trying hard enough. • They won't miss you if you are not here. • They'll like me if I try harder. • The things they say are right about me. • This relationship is going to fail because of me.

she experienced which she came to refer to as her Wise Woman speaking. She asked to take the Wise Women list of her and left behind Perfections list.

Handbooks

Handbooks[2] go hand in hand with co-created lists. One handbook that sits in the waiting room at my office is The Big Book of Worry Critters, Creatures, and Varmints. The inside cover reads:

> Welcome to the Big Book of Taming & Training Worry Critters, Creatures, and Varmints. This book is a growing collection of the ways children and youth handle 'Worry' when it becomes unruly, too big, or just takes up too much of their time.

The book is full of lists of ideas children have shared with me to assist with taming or training Worry Critters. These lists reflect their own know-how that became visible in our externalizing of Worry as an entity in need of training and taming. The children and youth take a copy of their plan and ideas with them but are also thrilled to contribute to the book in the hope their ideas will inspire other children. Other additions to the handbook include pictures of these worry creatures rendered visible by the children. From Worry Bats to Two Headed Worry Critters, to Hyenas and more obscure monsters, I have a diverse and useful collection of species and ideas.

Another handbook I've found very useful is titled the Manual for Young Care Givers. Originally, the manual was co-developed with a youth who had stepped into the position of providing significant care to her father following his diagnosis with diabetes and subsequent amputations of a limb because of the disease.

She came to the walk-in experiencing distress related to the isolation and stress she was experiencing in her care-giving role. Our discussion unearthed her exceptional "care giving abilities" and the lessons she learned through such a moving and very difficult experience. The inside of her manual reads:

> All young care givers live an apprenticeship of sorts. We are growing important skills! This manual shares those skills and learnings as well as even the hazards along the way on this precious journey!

Within the manual are some of her teachings, including "good days can turn into bad days in seconds, but remember, bad days can turn into great days just as quickly". Several other teachings accompany this idea.[3]

My waiting room is full of different handbooks covering diverse subjects including how to make friends with the scary night stuff (handling dark shadowy figures and voices at night), what to do when tornadoes come (a book about living with a sibling with severe FASD), calmness dances (for handling anger and frustration), and ways to get through the split up (manuals for kids navigating separation and divorce).

Statement of Position Documents

When people are invited to explore the effects of the problem in the various domains of their life, they enter a space of reflection and review. It creates a space within which they can consider their actions and choices and the effects of them on their relationships. They can consider how others are coming to know them. Within these conversations, sometimes people come to see the effects of the problem in a new light. They begin to shift their relationship with the problem.

For instance, in conversations about addiction, people may come to be far more acquainted with the effects of a drug habit in their life and relationships. Within these conversations, a "statement of position document" (White, 1995, p. 205) highlighting this turning point may prove useful in several ways.

A statement of position document reflects the emerging new position and notes a commitment to a new path. I invite people to co-craft these documents as a means to highlight their new commitment to a different path or course in life. I encourage them to make this public and invite them to identify people they will share the testament with.

> The time has come to make a change. I had not realized it was all an illusion. I think I am on top in the drug life but today the curtain came down. I am hurting the people I love and who care about my future, not just the moment. I am going to jail one day or will die if I don't turn this around. Today marks

the start of a new and important path. It is a step. I will need help. But this step will lead to a walk and eventually a run to the life I want, to the life I deserve. I can do this!

Statements of position can be embedded within broader next steps or action plans. They mark a turning point in a person's life. For some, this will be hard to sustain. Regardless, it marks a moment of clarity and effort that can be revisited in future conversations should they return to the walk-in.

Poems

I meet many people who have researched the internet collecting poems and sayings relevant to their circumstances. Together, poems[4] can be co-crafted, drawing from their own words, meaningful phrases, or expressions recorded on the conversation summary. Often, youth are very generous in allowing these poems to be circulated to others.

Break up Letters

Another style of take-away document I have found quite useful and quick to co-craft within a single session is the break-up letter. The person is invited into co-crafting this kind of documentation following an externalizing conversation. Externalizing conversations implicitly discuss the person as in relationship with the problem rather than the person as the problem. Separate from the problem but in relationship implies the relationship can be ongoing and yet adjusted, revised, or ended.

This conversation invites personal agency (the idea that they can do something) to the forefront as they outline actions to take to alter their relationship. Crafting the letter in itself is taking immediate action to alter the relationship, render it more visible and available for scrutiny. It is an agency enhancing activity. After asking permission to craft this kind of document and sharing my reasons for such an idea, I begin by addressing the problem. As we proceed, I gesture to the person/people consulting me to offer their ideas, inviting them to step into the co-authorship of the document.

The structure of this document is informed by Whites' Narrative Therapy Maps 1 and 2 (White, 2007). The first part of the letter is informed by Map 1 and covers the influence of the problem in the person's life. It draws out a characterization of the problem, a name for the problem, and invites exploration of the effects of the problem and people's evaluation of those effects. I then transition to exciting material from Map 2 after introducing and highlight a turning point. I draw out information about the person's influence over the problem. This includes the ways they counter the problem, defy it, undermine it, and live their life in preferred ways.

A. Address the letter to the problem.

"Dear Depression"
"Dearest Worry"
"Hello Sticky Thinking"
"Self-hate I have something I want to say to you"
"Dear Mother Blame"

B. Note how hard/easy it might be to break up with the problem.

"This is not easy for me to write but…"
"I am so excited to get rid of you…"
"I should have done this long ago…"
"This is so hard to say, but it's for the better of us both."
"I'm bouncing and not looking back…"

C. Outline the problems intentions, treatment, and strategies it uses to affect the life of the protagonist. This information is consistent with Map 1. Externalizing Conversations Map by Michael White (2007).

"I am sick and tired of your lies to try to get me to (think/feel/ act)…"
"Being with you is ruining my life…"
"I hate the way you try to…"
"At your worst, you…"

D. Highlight the turning point in the relationship in which the subject begins to see through, suspect, gain a clearer perspective on the problem and what the current relationship with the problem is doing to their life. Note, it is the current relationship with the problem that is problematic, not the problem itself. Some problems may be useful in terms of reminders, warning bells, and be helpful in certain situations. We don't want to erase the problem, but rather shift the relationship or domination of the problem.

"However, as I look at our relationship, I am clear that you must go."
"Now I am seeing through your lies…"
"Although it pains me, I want to take my life in a different direction.'
"Although it is scary and entering the unknown, I am…"

E. Highlight the ideas, strategies, ways, etc. that the person plans to adjust the relationship with the problem. This material is informed by Map 2.

"So, I am ending this relationship by…"
"I will be okay because I know that I am…"
"I'm making this happen, like it or not, by…"

F. You can state what the person might miss about the relationship, memories they'll keep with them, or what they learned from it that they will keep with them. We want to guard against totalizing problems, though. As in any relationship, whether it has been toxic, hot, or cold, sometimes the relationship was perhaps useful in some way. This may include a situation in which a problem assisted a person to keep themselves safe in the face of assault or lessened the effects of trauma. These kinds of problems may take the form of what authorities may call depression, worry, dis-association, avoidance. Although those problems served a purpose at a certain time in certain situations, they may no longer be necessary as people move their lives forward or are no longer in the threatening, assaultive context. For this reason, it's useful to acknowledge the helpfulness of the problem in the past and then highlight how it has been outgrown or is no longer working for the person given their more recent circumstances.

"Even though I know this is the best thing for me, I'll miss…"
"I'll always remember how you helped me out of those tough times, but we have outgrown each other."
"I've learned from our time together that…"
"This relationship has taught me…"
"I will miss how you kept me company when…"

G. Highlight the benefits of this breakup. This is wild speculation of a life less dominated by the relationship with the problem. You can speculate about the difference in significant domains of life-social, family, education, work, community.

"I know this will make my life more…"
"Being freer of our relationship will help me to…"
"As I move on, I can't wait to…"
"It's exciting to know that one day I'll be able to…"

This person's letter to OCD served as a starting place to reclaim their life from the tyranny of what had been labeled obsessive compulsive disorder.

Dear OCD,

The time has come for some changes around here. For years, I have been living with your demands and threats. You exaggerate and lie to me all the time. You try to have me do things I don't want to do. You try to use fear to control me like I'm your puppet on a string. You think you can dictate my day, where I can go, and who I can be around. Well, today I am cutting the strings and will be in charge of my own life. I understand how and why you came into my life. It was for a good reason. However, I am now safe and cared about and have things I need to do. So here is what's going to happen.

If you try to speak, I won't listen. In fact, I will do the opposite of what you say. If you make me uncomfortable, I will breathe you out of my body. I know being uncomfortable means I am growing. If you go on repeat, I will change the channel like switching from CNN to Friends. I will think about the things I like. I will remind myself I am safe, I am cared about, and I am growing my life.

I know this will be a big change for you and for me too, but it's about the future I want! That future begins today. I am no longer your puppet.

Sincerely,...

Certificates/Diplomas

We can craft specific certificates or diplomas on the spot as markers of new or revised meanings. For instance, I may craft a certificate awarded for taking a

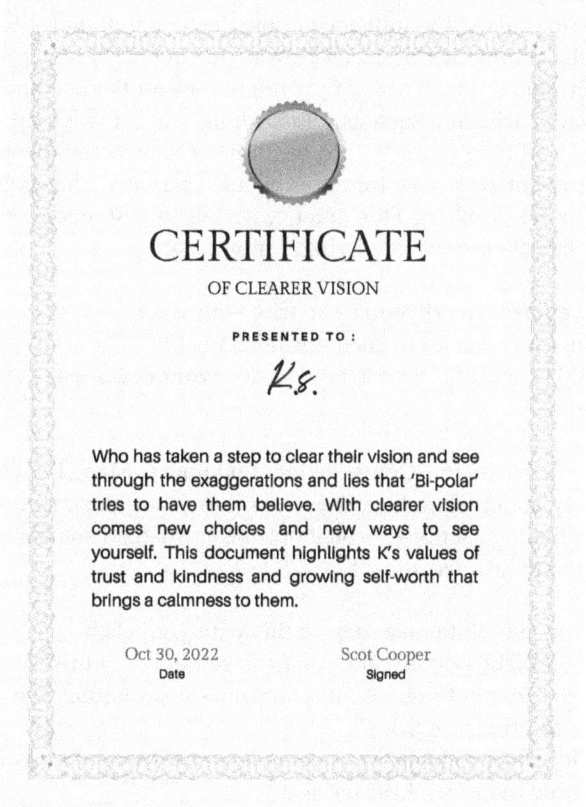

Figure 8.1 Sample certificate marking a shift in vision; from how the external-ized problem of bi-polar diagnosis would have them know them-selves in negative ways to a clearer view of the importance of trust and kindness in their life opening new options for living.

new position on a problem or to mark a renewed commitment to action. I may co-craft a diploma highlighting a person's knowledge to elevate it and bring it to the foreground. A certificate might highlight new learnings, beginnings of a project or a significant realization in the session. In some situations, I may induct a youth into various clubs, such as the Secret Society of Young Protesters or the Young Caregivers Club and award a certificate of membership. This serves to break the isolation that problems often benefit from.

Consulting the Documents and Speculating

As a brief narrative therapist, I am always looking for ways to foster conversation endurance, so stories-in-the-making become resistant to assimilation back into the problem story. White (1995) has proposed questions to foster endurance by eliciting from people their ideas about when to review their document as well as their predictions about the influence of the document in their life.

Following the completion of the take-away document, I invite people to identify the circumstances under which they might consult the document. At times, they may create a schedule such as, "First thing when I wake up, before each class at school and then twice before bedtime." Other times, people decide to read their document on a less formal schedule, perhaps whenever they sense vulnerability to the problem. This practice serves to help people contextualize the document into their everyday living. I might ask:

- How many copies would you like to take with you?
- Where would it be useful to keep this document?
- When would be a useful time to read/review your document so that it has the most influence?

Similar to the steps of the Conversation Endurance Map, I invite people to speculate wildly about what difference consulting their document will make in their thoughts/feelings/actions throughout the most relevant domains of their life, including to their sense of self.

- What difference will it make to have this with you when you leave?
- What might it make possible for you to be reminded of this information?
- What will this remind you about who you are becoming that the Problem would want to blind you from?
- What will it be like to know your document is helping other youth and families who come to our walk-in service?

Third, I invite the people to identify others with whom it would be important to share this document and how might those named respond. This serves to recruit an audience to the project who may witness and respond in meaningful ways. Inviting speculation about those responses paints a picture favourable to preferred outcomes. This serves to further counter and eventually displace the problem story.

- Who would be most important to share this document with when you leave here?
- How might they respond when you share this with them? Do you suppose they too would want to join you in this project?
- How will this shape how they are coming to know you?

Once the audience is identified, I supply participants with the requested number of copies for distribution. As noted, people are often also very willing to leave a copy behind that can be displayed in our waiting room to assist others who may experience similar circumstances.

Closing

Discovering ways to extend the influence of a single session remains a creative and important project. Take-away documents co-crafted during the single session conversation with the people consulting to us provide a meaningful vehicle for this effort. These documents informed by peoples' own know-how, skills, and preferences serve as keepsakes, foregrounding their ideas in creative and contextually relevant ways. When shared more broadly, take-away documents can contribute meaningfully to others who may experience similar circumstances.

Notes

1 This practice is inspired by the Consulting Your Consultants practice as shared by Michael White and David Epston, see Epston & White, 1990; Epston, White & 'Ben', 1995. We have several documents in our waiting room that archive the insider knowledge of past participants with the intent to share with others to hopefully make a difference in their lives. Through this process people may arrive seeking help but leave knowing they are helping others. This fosters a significant migration of identity within a single session.

2 The co-creation of handbooks is shared in chapter seven of *Playful Approaches to Serious Problems: Narrative therapy with children and their families* (Freeman, Epston & Lobovits, 1997, p.125–142). This is a wonderful and rich book of ideas and practices relevant to SST. Creating handbooks has become a useful brief narrative practice with young and old alike as a means to collect and circulate success stories and counter-problem ideas.

3 See the article Co-crafting Take-home Documents at the Walk-in (Cooper & 'Ariane', 2018) for the details of this document.

4 See Penwarden, S. (2020) for an account of what she terms the thera-poetic practice of co-crafting rescued-speech poems. Christopher Behan (2003) has also introduced some guidelines for this practice.

References

Behan, C. (2003). Rescued speech poems: Co-authoring poetry in narrative therapy. Retrieved from https://narrativeapproaches.com/resources/narrative-therapy-archive/345-2/

Cooper, S. & 'Ariane' (2018). Co-crafting take-home documents at the walk-in. In M.F. Hoyt, M. Bobele, A. Slive, J. Young & M. Talmon (Eds.), *Single-session therapy by walk-in or appointment: Clinical, supervisory, and administrative aspects.* New York: Routledge.

Epston, D. & White, M. (1990). Consulting your consultants: The documentation of alternative knowledges. *Dulwich Centre Newsletter*, 4, 25–35. Republished in D. Epston & M. White (1992), *Experience, contradiction, narrative and imagination: Selected papers of David Epston & Michael White, 1989–1991* (pp. 11–26). Adelaide, Australia: Dulwich Centre Publications.

Epston, D., White, M. & 'Ben', (1995). Consulting your consultants: A means to the co-construction of alternative knowledges. In S. Friedman (Ed.), *The reflecting team in action: Collaborative practice in family therapy* (pp. 277–313). New York: Guilford Press.

Freedman, J. & Combs, G. (1996). *Narrative therapy: The social construction of preferred realities.* New York. W.W. Norton.

Freedman, J. & Combs, G. (2002). *Narrative therapy with couples… and a whole lot more! A collection of papers, essays and exercises.* Adelaide: Dulwich Centre Publications.

Freeman, J., Epston, D. & Lobovits, D. (1997). *Playful approaches to serious problems: Narrative therapy with children and their families.* New York. W.W. Norton.

Korman, H. (2005). Harry's magic square. In T. S. Nelson (Ed.), *Education and training in solution-focused brief therapy* (pp. 89–90). Haworth Press.

Penwarden, S. (2020). Developing a thera-poetic practice: Writing rescued speech poetry as a literary therapy. *The International Journal of Narrative Therapy and Community Work*, (2), 44–53.

White, M. (1995). *Re-authoring lives: Interviews & essays.* Dulwich Centre Publications.

White, M. (2000). Re-engaging with history: The absent but implicit. In M. White, *Reflections on narrative practice: Essays & interviews* (pp. 35–58). Adelaide: Dulwich Centre Publications.

White, M. (2007). *Maps of narrative practice.* New York: W.W. Norton.

White, M. & Epston, D. (1990). *Narrative means to therapeutic ends.* New York: W.W. Norton.

Young, K., Dick, M., Herring, K. & Lee, J. (2008). From waiting lists to walk-in: Stories from a walk-in therapy clinic. *Journal of Systemic Therapies*, 27(4), 23–39. https://doi.org/10.1521/jsyt.2008.27.4.23

Chapter 9

Leave-Behind Documents

While the creation of take-away documents is a common practice in SST, occasionally, we also co-create what I refer to as leave-behind documents. Often these documents emerge out of externalizing conversations in which the Problem becomes more visible and merits spatial and social separation. Documents can take many forms, such as drawings of the Problem, lists of its haunting utterances, or even physical creations representing the Problem.

Starting the "leaving behind" involves entering a broader ceremony of sorts including verbal, imaginative, and physical separation from the Problem. It also involves a perceived shift in status from oppressed by the Problem to that of liberation and activism. That is, I invite people to enact separation in the physical world by placing the objectified Problem into a containment device at my office. Further, I invite them to leave behind the status associated with Problem domination. They are invited to take on and experiment with the revised status that comes with leaving the single session knowing the Problem remains with me, contained, and housed along with other peoples' Problems that have been left here for safekeeping.

Participation in this ceremony involves action by the person towards the Problem they have identified. Within the ceremony, people experience a sense of personal agency in that they are taking action to address the Problem and as such are directing their life. This experience of personal agency can ripple out into their real life informing an understanding that they *can* do something about the Problem, and they are no longer in servitude to its every command.

The Ceremony consists of four parts: rendering visible, separation, containment, and leaving behind. I'll illustrate these parts through a story of a 9-year-old young person I met.

Julia was brought to the walk-in by her mother out of concern that she was having trouble swallowing food since a severe choke episode on cheese from a pizza slice weeks earlier. Since that event, she was scared to eat and struggled to swallow food or drink water. She had seen the doctor and been cleared of any physical causes to her choking.

DOI: 10.4324/9781003431688-10

As is our usual practice, Julia had been offered a snack and water when she arrived. She tried to enjoy this snack but gagged and choked trying to swallow. I met Julia through her competencies, but when we transitioned to discuss the problem, she began to gag and choke again. She tried to sip water to help. It seemed the more we talked about the Problem the more it had a grasp of her. Our leave-behind document and containment ritual were what could be called a moment of single session desperation. I was unsure how to proceed as it seemed any way we tried to talk about what was going on, the Problem took Julia over.

It started to send fear thoughts my way, having me realize I was making things worse. At least this was until I heard about her mother's amazing chocolate cake that Julia really wanted to be able to eat at her birthday party that was scheduled in two weeks. We were determined to find a way to enjoy that cake. To start from a place of safety and with what Julia was most familiar with, I gathered an extensive history of her experience with eating her mom's chocolate cake. When was her first memory of tasting such a yummy cake? Did it come in layers? What was in-between the layers? Who else had enjoyed this with her? What was it like for her mother to know how much she enjoyed her baking?

To get away from the verbal, in contrast to talking about the cake, I invited Julia to visualize and draw a picture of the Problem imagining it as a critter trying to keep her from enjoying her birthday cake. Drawing the Problem seemed to help as Julia could start to make it visible with no choking or gagging. This was a clue to try out the leave-behind ceremony. It begins by entry into an externalizing conversation.

Rendering Visible

The person is first asked to render the Problem more visible, whether that be through a drawing, listing its tactics and tricks, or sculpting it with material.

"Julia, I understand that this Problem that everyone is calling anxiety has been messing with you and tries not to let you eat without choking and gagging. I wonder if you could draw me a picture of it so I could get to know it better? Can you picture it in your minds' eye? Give it a shape? Think about what colour it would be? Does it have eyes or ears or a mouth? Does it take up the whole page or only a little part? Once you have a picture in your mind, can you go ahead and draw it on this paper?"

Julia went straight to work, rendering the Problem visible. "What kind of talk comes out of its mouth?" I asked. She recounted several fear-based thoughts, like "It will happen again," "You're going to choke," and "You will die." Julia wrote these threats down on paper. Now, with a visual representation of the Problem, it was time to put some distance between Julia and It.

Separation

I introduced the notion that they have the option to then leave this Problem with me. They do not have to take it home with them where it has been messing with their life.

"Did you know you are welcome to leave that Problem here with me? You don't have to take it home with you! I'd be happy to keep it here with a lot of other kids Problems that they have entrusted me to keep safely contained so that they are not a bother anymore."

At this point, I show them to the containment canister that sits on the very top shelf in my office, away from anyone who could inadvertently release them from their realm. My current containment device is a bright orange cylindrical time capsule container that I have repurposed, modified, and converted into a containment device for all sorts of Problems with many different powers. I specially crafted it to foil any attempt by Problems to escape. The most risk is incurred when adding a new Problem as we must open the lid. That requires special instructions.

"Okay, Julia, I'm going to invite your mom to help us out here because sometimes they get difficult when we are about to capture a new Problem," turning my look to her mother, "Beth, can you help me hold this and please hold it tightly?"

As Beth takes hold, the canister starts to shake and wobble. It jumps and lurches, pulling both of us, but we keep our grip. Julia's eyes widen in surprise and intrigue. "Maybe we should shake this a bit to settle them down. It won't hurt them but will just settle them a bit."

Sometimes this can also be achieved by singing to them. Beth and I give the container a shake and I offer a breath of relief as they seem quieter. I go on to explain that Beth and I will loosen the top by unscrewing it to the point just before it is ready to come off. At that point, we will alert Julia to get ready to quickly place the Problem into the container as we pop the lid off and back on. Julia nods her understanding, and we are ready.

"Wait!", I exclaim. "I almost forgot the most important part!" I invite Julia to give every last bit of fear back to the Problem. I instruct her to fold the drawing tightly, as tight as she can, and then hold it gently to her forehead. "Okay, now think as hard as you can and send the fear thoughts back to the Problem." She visibly tightens her closed eyes. I can tell she is pushing the thoughts back on the Problem and I note this out loud. "When you are done thinking the fear thoughts and you see in your minds' eye, the last fear thought go back into the Problem, let us know by opening your eyes. We will count to three, open the containment and you must quickly put it in, okay?"

Julia nods and clenches her eyes even tighter. Seconds pass by that feel like a very long time till her eyes flick open. It's now our turn.

Containment

Once an act of separation is complete, it is time to contain the Problem. The method I use is to encourage the participation of all involved. Together, we open the device and the person holding the Problem places it within.

At this point Beth and I begin to unscrew the lid to the point it's almost completely undone. This helps to build anticipation. Together, Beth and I count to three, quickly remove the lid and Julia deposits the Problem. Immediately following the lid is placed and locked. The container shakes one last time as though wrestling with us until the Problem seems to settle into its fate.

Leaving Behind

Upon securing the Problem, I then place the device back in its safe place as a visual representation of the distance increasing between the person and the Problem.

"Here Julia, take the container and give it a shake. Can you hear it in there with the other Problems? How do you think we did; did we get it in there fast enough?" She nods a definitive yes, shaking the container while listening to the Problems bounce up and down. "Okay then, let's put it back up high on the shelf and I have just a few more questions to ask you if that is okay?"

I didn't see or hear from Julia and her mother again after that meeting until two years later. They had returned to the walk-in for another reason, and we recognized each other right away in the waiting room. I asked, "Whatever happened when you left, did you enjoy your cake?" Julia responded with a head nod, yes, and Beth added that when they left that night, it was no longer an issue.

This practice draws upon creativity, imagination, play, and drama to engage people in the experience of separating from externalized problems. It's a powerful activity, and I have had many visitors alongside colleagues brought to my office to take part in the ceremony.

Chapter 10

Externalizing Conversations

The creational aspect of language unlocks many novel and exciting ways to talk about the problems people experience. Externalizing conversations as an example of the creational feature of language help to render problems visible, sometimes as imaginary entities, that can be acted upon, trained, or taught by the person whose life they have come into. "Externalizing[1] is an approach to therapy that encourages persons to objectify and, at times, to personify the problem that they experience as oppressive" (White & Epston, 1990, p. 38). It would be hard to talk about brief narrative single session therapy without mention of externalizing conversations. I engage people in these kinds of conversations often. This happens for many reasons. They are a way to quickly enter novel conversations that introduce people to new ways to view their situation and expose proposals for action previously not considered. They quickly capture people's attention and interest as we look at experiences from a new angle. Externalizing conversations also help to shift away from blame and shame that people experience when they see themselves as the problem. At times, these conversations are like playful adventures as ideas and actions are linked in new and engaging ways. As you explored Chapter 8 you saw how these conversations also translate easily into various kinds of take-away documents.

Externalizing is not a technique but rather a practice evolving from a way of thinking about problems informed by post-structuralist ideas. Moving away from viewing problems as the result of structural deficiencies or pathologies located within the make-up of a person, externalizing is based on the assumption the person is not the problem, the problem is the problem. Externalizing conversations locate problems external to bodies as products of culture and history that have been socially constructed over time. As such, people are in relationship with Problems[2] and experience distress as Problems become oppressive of their lives and relationships.

Externalizing conversations use the creational aspect of language to the fullest as the practice involves a linguistic shift that breaks from usual ways of talking about problems by turning adjectives used to describe people into nouns that have an influence on people.

DOI: 10.4324/9781003431688-11

- "I'm so depressed I just can't see a way out of this!" becomes "Is Depression blinding you from a picture of how your future could be?"
- "It's just terrifying if I don't check the door 15 times!" becomes, "Has Fear become the boss of your life setting unrealistic rules for you?"
- "My life is like living a big storm all the time!" becomes "What are the ways you weather the Storms when they come?"

In this linguistic shift, the Problem is made visible, objectified, and held up for examination and scrutiny. Space is created to not only hear about and acknowledge what people have been through but to also hear about the ways people counter Problems in their lives through counter thoughts, feelings, and actions. Over the years I have been introduced to many species of Problems and the creative ways people reclaim their lives from them. These conversations begin a process wherein people can come to know themselves in more preferred ways, come to know they can affect the problem and liberate their lives from longstanding constraints.

In review of his work and as a means to teach the facilitation of these conversations, Michael White distilled his practice into two externalizing conversation maps. These are overly simplified groupings of the kinds of questions that shape externalizing conversations. The maps serve to assist the therapy to progress, providing what Michael later referred to as a scaffold for the conversation. As a scaffold, the questions in each domain assist people to link and connect experiences in useful ways. They help to grow the meaning of events and the conversation to get somewhere it would not have otherwise. It is a temporary structure for the conversation that falls away, becoming no longer needed as the story-in-the-making grows and takes hold.

The first map, Map 1. The Externalizing Conversations Map also known as the Statement of Position Map is concerned with exploring the influence of the Problem on the life of the person. It provides entry into these conversations inviting, first, the characterization and naming of the problem. I typically spend the most time in the first stage of this map. Often people will describe the problem in stock plot ways, so I take a considerable amount of time, when needed, to invite them to mentor me in the everyday experience of the problem and to ascribe a name to the Problem in their own voice rather than someone else's. I am seeking what White calls experience near descriptions. For instance, someone might say they have ADHD so I might ask questions such as:

- Tell me more about what you mean by that?
- What specifically do you do when this ADHD is around?
- Who came to give It that name?
- If you could give this problem a name of your own, what would you call it?

Suppose they were to call it the "band or circus playing in my head" I would proceed using their own words and metaphors. I might ask:

- What's it like having a band or a circus playing in your head?
- Is it a difficult thing or not too difficult?
- When it gets loud what difficulty does it make?
- How do you quiet the band or circus playing?

The second domain of inquiry invites people to map the effects of the Problem's activities across life domains such as home life, work, school, peer contexts, relationships with others/oneself, on hopes, aspirations, values, or future possibilities. These kinds of questions assist people to begin making links and connections between the Problem's activities and its influence on their life. In this domain I might ask:

- What's it like for you when this problem is around?
- What does it have you doing/thinking/feeling?
- What has it done to your relationships?
- How does IT have you treating yourself?
- What picture of you do you suppose it is giving people?
- What effects has IT had on your social life/ at school?

It is through inquiry about the effects of the Problem's activities on people's lives that people have opportunity to reflect on the Problem's influence. This may begin the revision of their position towards the Problem. For some, this is a very new conversation so we may explore effects thoroughly. For others, they are well acquainted with the effects of the Problem so we don't need to spend a great deal of time exploring, we can move on. I pay careful attention to and check in about how people experience these questions as, at times, too much exploration can be experienced as demoralizing. As noted previously, enacting our relational ethics has us continually paying attention to the possible effects of our practices on shaping people's experiences.

The third domain of inquiry has people consider the effects of the Problem, evaluate them, and draw learnings, realizations, or conclusions about what has been happening. It is in this phase that people establish their position on the Problem. Often, people have not had opportunity to have this kind of conversation. As they explore and evaluate the effects of the Problem, they may come to experience a new or revised attitude towards it. In this domain I might ask:

- What is that like for you and your family, a good thing or not so good?
- Is this a positive development or negative or something in-between?
- Does this move your life closer to how you want it to be or farther from that picture?
- Is that something you would like more or less of?
- Do you think that is the way it should be?

The fourth domain of inquiry asks people to justify their evaluation of the effects of the problem eliciting the context that informs their evaluations. This brings forward concepts related to people's intentions for their life, values they hold on to, or ideas about a preferred identity. Questions asked may include:

- Can you tell me a story about your life that would help me understand your position on this?
- Why do you feel this way about the Problem?
- Why do you want this to change?

These four categories of inquiry assist people to reflect on the Problem from a different vantage point inviting linking and connecting to the events of their lives. As noted, it not only provides the entry into an externalizing conversation but also can assist people to revise their position on the problem as a result of such review. Not only may they come to see they need to do something about the Problem, but they might also come to see they *can* do something in contrast to when they arrived suffering under it's influence.

Figure 10.1 represents the progression of questions in four categories and is read from the bottom to the top. Adopting a Vygotskian influence, White noted how the questions assist people to distance from what they know and know how to do (the known and familiar) moving towards what's possible to know and do in the real world. Although the map moves from the bottom to the top, it's not intended to present the work in linear and scripted ways. Therapeutic conversations are much messier than a teaching device and at any point we weave into other maps and then back. They assist us to not lose our way in conversation, to remain aware of the intention of our questions even when the content of the conversation becomes evocative or difficult to navigate.

While Map 1 explores the experience of the Problem, we do not typically want to dwell there. That conversation, for some, can be difficult and at worst further demoralizing. Working within a time constraint I do not want to leave people mired within an account of the influence of the Problem on their life and it is our responsibility to monitor for and check in about when enough of this kind of conversation has been had. Many times, natural transitions towards people's influence on the Problem can be heard and followed up upon. They may be heard in expressions such as, "It hasn't always been like this", or "That's not my usual self, I know it's just the depression". These expressions provide openings into storylines about the ways people resist or counter Problems. As a guide, White developed Map 2, the Externalizing Conversations Map.

Externalizing Conversations Map 2 seeks to learn about the influence of the person on the life of the Problem. The understanding that all people resist problems, respond to them in some way, and take actions in the face of Problems informs Map 2. The categories of questions elicit unique outcomes, exceptions,

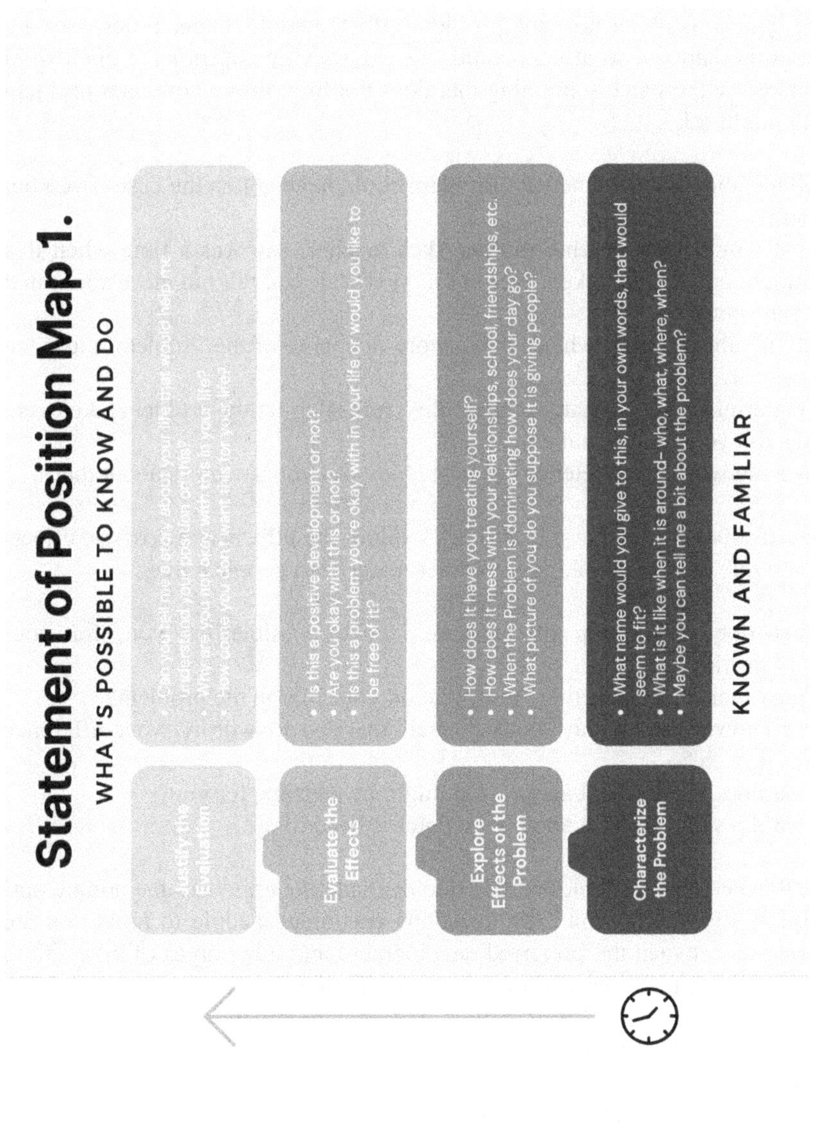

Statement of Position Map 1.

WHAT'S POSSIBLE TO KNOW AND DO

Justify the Evaluation
- Can you tell me a story about your life that would help me
- Understand your position on this?
- Why are you not okay with this in your life?
- Have some you don't want this for your life?

Evaluate the Effects
- Is this a positive development or not?
- Are you okay with this or not?
- Is this a problem you're okay with in your life or would you like to be free of it?

Explore Effects of the Problem
- How does it have you treating yourself?
- How does it mess with your relationships, school friendships, etc.
- When the Problem is dominating how does your day go?
- What picture of you do you suppose it is giving people?

Characterize the Problem
- What name would you give to this, in your own words, that would seem to fit?
- What is it like when it is around– who, what, where, when?
- Maybe you can tell me a bit about the problem?

KNOWN AND FAMILIAR

Figure 10.1 Externalizing Conversations Map adapted from White, M. (2007, 2012).

initiatives and infuse them with significance through linking and connecting with other developments, values, hopes, or intentions for life. The procession of questions invites people to characterize an initiative, unique outcome or exception, at times assigning a name and then exploring the effects of the preferred development. As noted, sometimes unique outcomes "pop up" in the process of asking questions about how the problem affects people. Other times they are found in the gaps; in what is not said. We ask specific questions to elicit from the person's experience something that does not fit with the dominant problem story. I might ask:

- Tell me about a time when the Problem could have gotten the best of you but didn't?
- What would your (friend, mother, dad, teacher) say was a time when this Problem could have taken over but didn't? Can you tell me more about that circumstance?
- Tell me about a time when you're more in charge of the Problem, more the boss of it.
- What might you call that; a step, ability, refusal to let the problem take over?
- How did you know to take that step?
- Does the word "competence" fit here? Yes, can you say more about that?

Similar to Map 1, together we can then explore the effects and possible effects of the unique outcome, linking it to other material in people's lives.

- What does that "step of self-care" make possible for you, for your relationships?
- What other effects has this "step" had on your life/on the problem?
- When you think that way about yourself, that you are worthy, what difference does it make?
- What does that suggest about what might be possible for you?
- What does that suggest about who you are becoming?

In the third category people are asked to evaluate the effects of the unique outcome, initiative, exception. The questions encourage people to reflect on the connections between the preferred development and other areas of their life to begin to draw realizations and learnings specific to them.

- Do you see this as an important step?
- Are these preferred developments?
- Is this a good thing, not a good thing, or somewhere in between?
- What are you realizing about what else is possible?
- What does that suggest about what you want for your life or is important to you?

Again, similar to Map 1, the fourth category has people speak to their justification for where they stand on these preferred developments. The questions have people formulate their ideas about life and identity relating the events to their intentions, values, and beliefs about the kind of life they are striving for. We may ask:

- Why is that an important step/preferred development?
- Why is that something you would want more of?
- How come you're taking this position?

Figure 10.2 provides a simplified visualization of Map 2. Again, it reads from the bottom to the top progressing from what people know and do towards what might be possible to know and do.

These maps are important to know thoroughly. They commonly inform SST conversations. A great deal has been written about externalizing conversations for you to study[3] and reference. I offer this vignette to demonstrate externalizing practice in a single session.

I had met Addison, an 8-year-old, one late afternoon at the walk-in. She settled at the waiting room blackboard drawing flowers and animals while her mother Gwen, completed the paperwork noting that Addy "probably has an anxiety disorder". They were seeking the services of a psychiatrist at the recommendation of the family doctor as they were contemplating seeking medication to help her. They had come to the walk-in hoping for "some ideas for Addy to handle her worries and the anxiety" while they waited for an appointment with the psychiatrist.

As noted, the pre-session questionnaire asks, "What would be most important to talk about today". Replies similar to Gwen's such as "to talk about my Depression", "how to cope with Anxiety", "ideas to help with ADHD", "ways to deal with my OCD", are common. Addy's introduction and these examples demonstrate how the language of pathology circulates freely amongst the population and comes to represent children and people in general. These answers are revealing of how the politics of culture are infiltrating the therapeutic context. They reflect how people have adopted medicalized understandings of experience in their everyday language whether they have been given the diagnosis or not. That understanding of their experience offers a limited range of responses and the naming of the distress as pathology begins to frame and shape the expression of the distress itself. Children, in particular, have little say to resist being defined in this way.

While the caregivers had been considering Addy's distress as a disorder, I was relieved that, at this point, it had not yet been affirmed by an authority. There was still opportunity to think and talk about her experiences differently; in a way that did not have the problem define her identity or render her as disordered. When people come to the walk-in defined by diagnosis to the point that it significantly

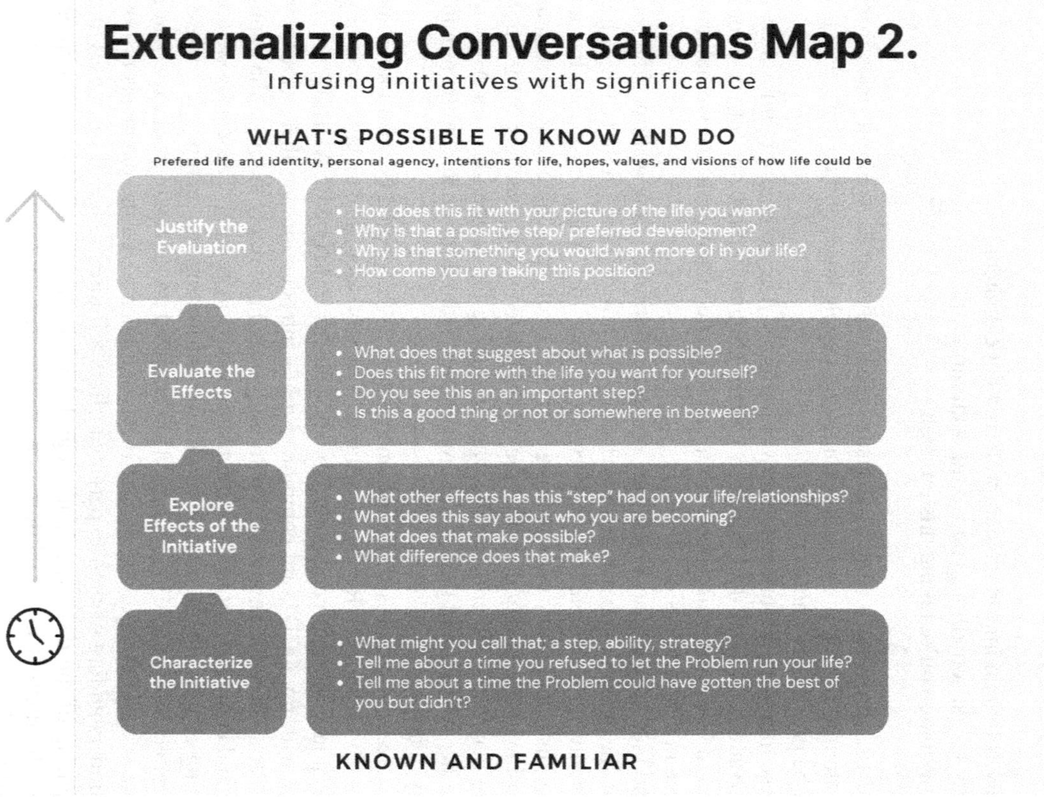

Externalizing Conversations Map 2.

Infusing initiatives with significance

WHAT'S POSSIBLE TO KNOW AND DO

Prefered life and identity, personal agency, intentions for life, hopes, values, and visions of how life could be

Justify the Evaluation
- How does this fit with your picture of the life you want?
- Why is that a positive step/ preferred development?
- Why is that something you would want more of in your life?
- How come you are taking this position?

Evaluate the Effects
- What does that suggest about what is possible?
- Does this fit more with the life you want for yourself?
- Do you see this an an important step?
- Is this a good thing or not or somewhere in between?

Explore Effects of the Initiative
- What other effects has this "step" had on your life/relationships?
- What does this say about who you are becoming?
- What does that make possible?
- What difference does that make?

Characterize the Initiative
- What might you call that; a step, ability, strategy?
- Tell me about a time you refused to let the Problem run your life?
- Tell me about a time the Problem could have gotten the best of you but didn't?

KNOWN AND FAMILIAR

Figure 10.2 Externalizing Conversations Map 2 adapted from White, M. (2007, 2012).

limits possibility, in those circumstances, I invoke a specific kind of external-izing conversation called a counter-story[4] discussed in the next chapter. For now though, Addy was experiencing distress, and it was yet to be specifically defined or fully come to represent her identity. Picking up from her paperwork the under-standing that the family was seeing Addy's distress as possibly a disorder, I was sensitive to the story of pathology that had already taken some hold. To mitigate this, an externalizing conversation seemed like it might be useful.

As our conversation began, I intentionally asked questions that helped me learn about Addy through stories of competence, about her many skills and won-derful qualities that her mother noticed about her. I learned how she and her parents' bred dogs. Addy demonstrated many skills related to the task and she told me about her own dog whom she had taught to do several tricks like shake a paw, lie down, and roll over. I commented on how this was such a wonderful way to meet Addy; to learn that she was a caregiver to pets and had skills in training the animals she cared about.

Transitioning the conversation to what would be most important for us to talk about, I learned how Addy had been having worries that their family was going to be killed and that these Worries were keeping her up late at night and even visited in her dreams.

Scot:	Can you teach me a bit more about the Worries? (This phras-ing begins to introduce a linguistic shift from adjective to noun and is a purposeful move away from the name Anxiety.)
Addy:	Thunderstorms.
Gwen (Mother):	When there is a thunderstorm, she thinks tornadoes are going to come and kill us all.
S:	Do the Worries try to mess with you in any other ways?
G:	They get her to check outside way too much or running to the window every 5 minutes thinking that robbers are com-ing. (Addy's mother has already shifted linguistically)
S:	Okay, so Worry tries to get you to think bad things are going to happen, are there other things It tries to get you to think? (Addy struggles to answer)
G:	I think she gets down on herself too. She's always saying nobody likes me or I have no friends, but she is always play-ing with friends so I'm not sure where that's coming from.
S:	(To Addy) What do you think about what your mom is say-ing? Does Worry get you thinking down about yourself or your friendships?
A:	(nods yes)
S:	Okay, can I ask a few more questions about this, about what it's like having Worries like these?
A:	(nods yes)

I sense this conversation is hard for Addy, perhaps she is experiencing shame, embarrassment, or my questions are just too complex at this point. I decide I need to return to her competencies and ask about experiences that are known and familiar to her.

S: Addison can you tell me something? Does your dog run around your house making messes everywhere like peeing on your things or chewing all your toys?

A: No. (a small smile)

S: No, well how come?

A: Because we trained him.

S: Oh, you trained him. How did you train him?

Addison steps a little more into the conversation within this more familiar territory of experience and takes me through all the ways she taught her dog to know where to go to the bathroom, how to shake a paw and lie down. Within this demonstration I am drawn to her technique.

S: Addison I heard that you… what did you call it … give commands. What do you mean by you give commands?

A: Like I tell him what to do.

S: You tell him what to do? And I noticed you used a different sounding voice when you showed me that, do you have to use a different voice?

A: A bossy voice.

S: Why is that?

A: Because I have to let him know I am the boss.

S: You have to let him know you are the boss? Why, what difference does that make?

A: Because then he knows I'm in charge and he will do what he is told.

S: Okay, and if he learns to do what he is told then he won't be making messes all over the place and will know what he can and can't do?

A: Yes, so he knows how to behave and is trained.

At this point I have had Addy mentor me in her skills and wisdom related to commanding and training her dog so that it doesn't make messes in her life. As a means to highlight this and further the externalizing conversation I use a short re-telling to springboard to my next questions.

S: Addy, I'm just thinking about what you have been teaching me about how you trained your dog to behave, and it had me wondering something. I was wondering if your Worry is a lot like your dog was when you got him. It's running around making messes in your life, gets noisy and annoying, and keeps you up all night. It doesn't know how to behave or that you are the boss. Do you suppose Worry could use some training like your dog did? Because imagine if you hadn't trained your dog! It would be messing all over the house and be hard to live with. So, do you suppose if we think about Worry as a creature or critter, that it could use some of your training?

Addy related to this idea so to further develop the concept I asked her to picture in her mind's eye what her worry critter would look like if she were to give it a shape or body and some characteristics like a mouth, eyes, ears, fur, etc. Once she had a good picture of it in her mind, I asked her if she could draw a picture of It so we could get to know it even better. Once her picture was complete, we explored its behaviour and effects of that behaviour further. Often, I will invite a physical rendering of the Problem either drawn, crafted with play-do, or selected from a group of paper monsters I have sitting out. This physical rendering assist people to step into the externalizing more easily.

S: I see your worry critter has a mouth; what kind of talk comes out of Worries mouth? (Continuing on Map 1, Addy is now able to more specifically share her experience near descriptions characterizing the Problem)

A: Like scary stuff like tornadoes are going to come and kill us all.

S: That doesn't seem very nice, what else?

A: The house is going to catch on fire, or my food is bad and if I eat it, I will die.

Having made the worry critter visible, Addy begins to share more from this different vantage point. I start to list these expressions and inquire further. Listing helps to organize the tactics of problems and provides a way to visibly contrast it to a counter list as the conversation progresses.

S: Okay, would it be okay if I get some of these things down on a list? The reason is if we know what Worry is up to in your life then it will make it easier to know what kind of training it needs. Would this be okay?

A: (Nods yes)

S: Okay so on this side of the paper I'll write, "Worry tries to have me think the house will catch fire, tornadoes will come, food is poisoned...". What else does Worry try to have you believe? (Continuing to characterize the Problem. Note the insertion of the word "try" implying It is not always successful)

A: Well sometimes it gets me thinking I have no friends or that nobody likes me so then I don't really want to go to school.

S: Do you get believing the things this worry tells you about yourself and the world?

A: Sometimes I start to believe it, but I also know it's not true.

This is an expression that catches my attention as a possible entry point into a story-in-the-making. It reflects a counter-knowledge and we are listening for these openings. Often, they are faint or go by very quickly, but when asked about, lead to creative and useful ideas about how to address problems.

S: You know it's not true?

A: Ya, but…

S: So, the things Worry often says aren't true? Are those like lies that It tries to tell you? Does this worry critter try to lie to you?

A: Yes, I guess so.

S: (Holding up the list for review) Okay, if you could give this side of the list a name, would that be a good name for it; The Worry That Lies to Me?

A: Yes, The Worry That Lies to Me!

S: Okay let me write that in for the title.

Having characterized the Worry, learning about some of Its tactics and effects of those tactics I move up Map 1 into inviting her to take a position on the effects/behaviour of Worry.

S: Well, what do you think about the worry critter's behaviour? Are you okay with It making messes in your life, lying to you, trying to scare you and even trying to stop you from going to school and enjoying friendships?

A: Nope, it's not behaving.

S: Okay, so do you suppose it's time to give It some training to show It you are the boss?

A: Ya, I could turn it into my pet. (At this point Addy is preparing to revise her relationship with the Problem. She has taken a position and made visible some of the tactics of the problem and linked them to the effects on her life.)

This moment provided an offshoot into Map 2 where we explored times when Addy had been more the boss of the Worry. Her mother shared some recent examples when she had played with her friends, free of the Worry Critters lies.

S: How were you able to do that, to keep Worry in its place so it didn't ruin your fun with your friends?

A: I just ignored it and had fun.

S: But that couldn't have been easy, what did you do when It tried to have you think of Its lies?

A: I didn't listen to it, I just had fun.

S: Okay, so what are you thinking differently when you are having fun that Worry wouldn't want you to be thinking.

A: I have friends, they like me, this is fun…

S: So, what do you call those thoughts? Are they like positive thoughts or… (This is back to the naming and characterization of the initiative)

A: Nice thoughts.

S: Ah, so thinking "nice thoughts" about yourself and your friends, is that one way you be the boss of Worry?

A: Yep!

I get permission from Addy to list this idea under the heading Ways to Be the Boss of Worry beside the list of Lies that Worry Tries to Tell. We then take some time exploring other ways that Addy had been more the boss of the Worry and continue to list these activities. She includes "Give It Commands" so It can learn to behave in the same way she gave commands to her dog. We write down some of these commands including "Be quiet", "Not now", and "Leave me alone". Addy demonstrates[5] for her mother and I these commands and the forceful tone required to show she is in charge. I always want to invite an attitude equal to or exceeding the attitude of the Problem and Addy has a very commanding voice when needed.

At this point, I feel we have enough material to begin to craft the training plan for the Worry Critter but out of curiosity I ask one more question situated in the characterization level of Map 1.

S: Addison, I'm just curious when did you notice Worry starting to really make messes in your life, like has it always been this poorly behaved or had it known you were the boss before and forgot?

M: Addy likes to watch the news, so I wonder if that might be feeding some of this?

S: What do you mean?

M: Well, I'm just thinking that maybe Worry feeds off of some of the things she sees on the news? Addy likes to watch CNN and news shows about things so…

S: Addy, what do you think about what your mom is saying? Do you think the Worry feeds off of bad news stories? Do you think that could be like unhealthy food for It?

A: Ya, it makes the Worry bigger?

S: So, if bad news stories are like unhealthy food for the Worry what kind of food do you think you should be feeding it?

It comes to light that the Worry Critter was becoming most unruly around the time Addy had been watching a show about natural disasters. Worry was using what had started as a general interest and turned it into unhealthy concern. Addy decides she should be feeding the Worry "good news stories" so that the Worry doesn't get too big.

In his later work and further influenced by Vygotskian thinking, Michael combined Maps 1 and 2 into the Scaffolding Conversations Map (White, 2007; Malinen et al., 2012). The Scaffolding Conversations Map is especially suited to single session conversations as he had added a fifth level to the maps that traditionally showed four levels. He referred to the fifth level as very high-level distancing from the known and familiar as it is specifically concerned with generating proposals for action and predicting the possible outcome of those actions.

For Addy, she had come up with several ideas that assisted her to be the boss of the Worry. Her final realization about the need to feed It good news stories came to be included in her take-away document and included in the Guidebook for Taming and Training Worry Critters, Creatures, or Varmints. She also included:

- Give It commands when It starts to become unruly in the night or when the weather gets stormy.
- Think nice thoughts about myself and my friends each day such as we have fun together and I am liked.

To generate this document, I asked questions like:

- What ideas should we write in here as part of your Worry Critters training?
- How often will you need to use these ideas?
- When would it be good to review this guidebook?
- Should we leave a blank page for you to write in new ideas as you discover what else works?
- When you are done training the Worry, how will you know?

Commiserate with the micro-skills in phase three of our process we then identified a period of practice for the training of Worry prior to consideration of the need for further services. An option often included is to return to the walk-in to revise the plan of action as often small revisions can make a difference assisting the ripples of change to continue.

I believe the family travelled a great distance in this conversation. When they arrived, they were considering her distress as an internally located disorder and seeking medication as an external control. Externalizing practice assisted us to come to know her differently. She had ways that she acted upon her distress with varying degrees of success. She was an active agent in rendering it visible and collaborating on how to further address it. She contributed to developing the guide for training the Worry. That practice, itself, is an act of personal agency in which Addy experienced being able to do something about this concern. Structuring practice after the session helped to further her efforts. The training ideas added to our larger collective document titled "The Manual for Training and Taming Worry Critters, Creatures and Varmints" sits in our waiting room as a resource to other people experiencing Worry in their lives. It has evolved into a large collection of ideas and practices.

There are a few points I want to highlight relevant to externalizing conversation and single session therapy.

Listening Highlights

The understanding of problems as external to people requires us to expand further the range of material we are listening for including:

1. Listen with the understanding that the Problem is separate from the person (Freedman and Coombs, 2002, p.28). It's a thing or entity influencing the person. I often think of the problem as a critter, creature or entity up to something in the lives of people. At times, it helps to get into the character of the Problem. Think as if you were the Problem. Consider what tactics you might use, what ideas might you endorse and circulate.
2. Listen for acts of oppression on behalf of the problem. A measure of the dominance of a Problem is reflected in how much airtime it gets in the story telling. We can listen for how It represents people in their story. Listen for how It defines them and the possibilities It eclipses through Its authority.
3. Listen for "it's ways"–coaching, blinding, lying, twisting, exaggerating, restricting, demanding, making rules, directing, stealing, misrepresenting, obscuring, tempting, silencing, threatening, etc. How does It go about doing its work?
4. Listen for gaps in the dominance of the Problem. This provides clues to counter thoughts, feelings and actions for further exploration.
5. Listen for the hopes, values, intentions, and preferences reflected in the GAPS of the problem's dominance.

Transitions

Entering into externalizing conversations in single session therapy presents, for many, a very different way of talking about their experiences. As we do not have the benefit of ongoing sessions for people to get used to the linguistic shift, it can be useful to transition to this way of speaking with a clear and transparent explanation of the process.

- "It sounds to me that for a long time you have thought of your distress as a flaw or dysfunction of yours. I'm wondering if we could have a different kind of conversation about this problem? What if we think about IT as a thing outside of you that you are up against? Perhaps it is trying to mess with you and your life? This might be a strange way to talk about it at first but the reason I'm wondering about this is because I'm hoping it opens up some different

possibilities for you. Would it be okay if we explore this way of thinking and talking about the problem for a bit?"
- "What if you think about this Problem as a thing, a critter, creature or entity? Can you picture it in your mind's eye? What shape might it have, what colour, what other features? Or, does it resemble an animal of some sort? Once you have an image of it in your minds eye, can you draw me a picture of it so we can get to know it?"

This transition and transparency about why we are suggesting talking in this way can assist people into the shift in mindset.

These are Important Identity Shaping Conversations

Externalizing conversations are conversations about identity as much as action. As noted in Chapter 2, we are always involved in identity projects in these conversations as identity is socially and relationally shaped. People come to know themselves through our responses. It is common for people to arrive at the walk-in with identity conclusions shaped by pathology. The discourse of pathology as become internalized as they locate the problem in their brain or structures of the mind. They may introduce themselves as Depressed, ADHD, Bi-polar, etc. They have not come to these conclusions on their own but rather through some social interaction, most often with another health professional. In that time, they have been ascribed what Goffman (1963) terms well as a 'spoiled identity'. The consequence of this can be to limit what is viewed as possible and possible to do. However, when the internalized discourse of problems is located outside of people and a protagonist/antagonist relationship is established, we are living a relational ethic, aware of and sensitive to the various potential constructions of identity within a therapeutic conversation that may unfold (Paré, 2014). In separating the person and the problem through talk, new space is created for the generation of novel or perhaps unseen ways to proceed in life. As problems come to no longer represent who the person is, new more preferred considerations of identity become possible.

These are Personal Agency Conversations

When problem discourse is internalized, meaning people think to themselves 'I am the problem', the way to attack the problem is to attack oneself such as seen with self-harm or through external controls such as pharmaceutical intervention. What becomes obscured in those circumstances is the idea of personal agency; the sense that a person can do something about the problem in their life, that they can direct their life and are not at the whim of their experiences.

Externalizing conversations make space for the experience of personal agency inviting participants to defy the problem, resist it, and alter their relationship with it in some way. These counter acts often go unnoticed or may be discounted in the face of influential and widely circulated internalized problem focused meta-narratives. We can be on the lookout for the ways people have resisted problems to foreground that material to bring into stories-in-the-making. In this practice the experience of personal agency is resuscitated. Resisting individualizing problems and supporting personal agency are acts of our relational ethics.

Common Mishaps

When entering into externalizing conversations under time constraint there are some common mishaps to watch out for.

1. Vanquishing problems: We are not trying to invite the idea that a problem should be completely vanquished from a person's life. We are inviting a revision of the relationship with the problem, reducing its influence, so that it is less oppressive in their life.
2. Mismatching the posture: It's useful to match the response of the person to how the problem is characterized. For instance, if the posture or influence of the problem is oppressive then match with language of liberation. If It is being unjust, the person may want to bring justice, if It is mis-informed, the person may want to educate the Problem. This assists the conversation to remain sensible and experience-near.
3. Introducing or prioritizing "contest" or "battle" metaphors: At times, metaphors such as "rage war against the problem" or to "beat down the problem" may emerge. I try to move away from violent metaphors to describe the changing relationship between the person and the problem. This is an intentional move away from the popular notion of using violence or aggression to solve problems. Instead, I may circulate revised language for this such as overcoming the problem, outwitting It, training It, etc.
4. Use of static definitions of the problem: It is important to elicit and listen for people's experience-near definitions and names for the problem. Listening with a static, stock plot idea about a problem can limit our curiosity. Avoid generalizations or asking questions from a canonized world view. Stay curious!
5. Settling on a name too early: Even in the time constraint of a single session it is important to take the time to elicit an experience-near name for the problem. A name that doesn't accurately capture one's experience may seem contrived.
6. Too loosely characterizing the problem: There is a balance needed in taking time to adequately characterize the problem with keeping a watch for the effect of the conversation on the person. Some may experience discussing the problem as demoralizing or the Problem may try to take them back in time to re-experience what they have been through. While we want to honour

what people have gone through and elicit their descriptions, we also have a responsibility for their safety. If problem talk becomes problematic, we need to move the conversation along, check in with them and transition to Map 2.

Within this chapter I have outlined the practice of externalizing conversations, a kind of conversation well suited to time constrained therapy as a means to enter novel ways to talk about people's experiences. New or previously discounted proposals for action are revealed. Further to this, I hope it becomes clear how externalizing conversations bring the social context of problems forward. People go through things. Their experiences are shaped by how those events are understood, how they are talked about, and by who gets to talk about them. Externalizing begins to question those limiting understandings or what has been understood as truth, opening cracks for revised meanings and revised identities.

Notes

1 For a thorough account of the practices of externalizing conversations see White and Epston, 1990, White, 2007, White, 2011.
2 The word 'problem' is capitalized to reflect the shift to addressing them as external entities.
3 See Young, K. (2008) *Narrative Practice at a Walk-in Therapy Clinic: Developing Children's Worry Wisdom*, for an excellent example of externalizing worry/anxiety in a single session.
4 A counter-story is a specific kind of story dedicated to rehabilitating a spoiled identity and directly counters the story of the problem. For a detailed account of counter story see Lindemann (2001) and for a practice example see my article Cooper, S. (2014). Brief narrative practice at the walk-in clinic: The rise of the counterstory [online]. *International Journal of Narrative Therapy and Community Work, 2*, 23–30.
5 I often invite performance of the skills as a means of rehearsal to assist the emerging story-in-the-making to be more durable.

References

Cooper, S. (2014). Brief narrative practice at the walk-in clinic: The rise of the counterstory [online]. *International Journal of Narrative Therapy and Community Work, 2*, 23–30.

Freedman, J. & Combs, G. (2002). *Narrative therapy with couples… and a whole lot more! A collection of papers, essays and exercises.* Adelaide: Dulwich Centre Publications.

Freeman, J., Epston, D. & Lobovits, D. (1997). *Playful approaches to serious problems: Narrative therapy with children and their families.* New York: W.W. Norton.

Goffman, E. (1963). *Stigma: Notes on the management of spoiled identity.* Engelwood Cliffs, NJ: Prentice Hall.

Lindemann Nelson, H. (2001). *Damaged identities, narrative repair.* Cornell University Press: New York.

Malinen, T., Cooper, S. J. & Thomas, F. N. (Eds.). (2012). *Masters of narrative and collaborative therapies: The voices of Andersen, Anderson, & White.* New York: Routledge.

Paré, D. A. (2014). Social justice and the word: Keeping diversity alive in therapeutic conversations. *Canadian Journal of Counselling and Psychotherapy 48*(3), 206–217.

White, M. (2007). *Maps of narrative practice.* W.W. Norton: New York.

White, M. (2011). *Narrative practice: Continuing the conversations.* W.W. Norton: New York.

White, M. (2012). Scaffolding a therapeutic conversation. In T. Malinen, S. J. Cooper, & F. N. Thomas (Eds.), *Masters of narrative and collaborative therapies: The voices of Andersen, Anderson, & White* (pp. 121–169). Routledge.

White, M. & Epston, D. (1990). *Narrative means to therapeutic ends.* New York: W.W. Norton.

Young, K. (2008). Narrative practice at a walk-in therapy clinic: Developing children's worry wisdom. *Journal of Systemic Therapies, 27*(4), 54–74.

Chapter 11

Counter-Storying in Single Session Therapy

While externalizing conversations provide a novel way of discussing problems and quickly expose new possibilities for addressing them, they also importantly provide opportunity to revise identity. Michael White often used to say we are always involved in identity projects in therapeutic conversations, meaning how we do what we do contributes to and shapes how people come to know themselves. He was calling for attention to how one comes to see themselves is socially and relationally shaped. It's a call to therapists to take responsibility for the effects of how we talk with people.

In SST, especially given the time constraint, it's important to foster conversations in which people will experience themselves in preferred ways and with a sense that they can direct their lives. However, many people arrive introducing themselves through a label or diagnosis that has been prescribed to them by an authority or worse yet self-prescribed. The discourse of pathology, that is, the medicalized descriptions and characterization of people's actions and experiences has come to define who they are and consequently what they see as possible or more so not possible for themselves. It is a cultural construction that has been internalized, accepted as the way it is, and thus has been unquestioned.

At times, I meet people who identify so strongly with their label that it's blinding new possibilities for their identity and lives. Some have been given the label at a very young age, a time with no possibility to protest the description of them. Others have experienced such influence by the authorities scribing the label that they dare not question what it suggests about them. The label has been so highly endorsed that it filters all further experience and forecasts an unchanging future. This can be heard in comments such as, "Well I've had depression for so long, it's hard to know anything else" or "I'm bipolar, so it's going to be like this for the rest of my life".

Yet, people come to the walk-in seeking relief from their experience of distress even though it may be unimaginable according to their medical files or the general opinion of others in their life. It is in these circumstances that it can be very useful to turn specifically to co-authoring "counter-stories" (Freeman, Epston & Lobovits, 1997; Lindemann, 2001; Ingamells, 2016) as a means to

DOI: 10.4324/9781003431688-12

rehabilitate identity and renew the possibility that people can take action and grow a more preferred life. It is through the process of counter-storying that counter-practices from local knowledges are foregrounded and come to inform action plans.

Counter-Stories

A counter-story is a specific kind of story purposefully evoked to directly counter a dominant internalized problem story and more importantly to rehabilitate a persons spoiled identity.[1] It directly counters identity claims propagated by the dominant discourse of the problem story. Counter-stories rise out of the gaps and inconsistencies of the problem story involving a plot in juxtaposition to the dominant problem narrative. In brief narrative therapy, they are woven together, response by response, into a storyline rendering the Problem as the antagonist in juxtaposition to the person as protagonist.

David Epston had introduced me to the work of Hilde Lindemann Nelson (2001) who details the influence of dominate narratives and the ingredients of an enduring counter-story. She highlights how a useful counter-story:

- Fills in details the dominant[2] narrative has left out, ignored or underplayed,
- Resists, addresses, and repairs the damage of identity caused by dominant narratives,[3]
- Are shared, recruiting others to witness and respond to revived preferred identity, and
- Invite new proposals for action as they resist dominant narratives.

Importantly then, "counterstories don't merely reflect a shift in understanding, they set out to cause a shift" (2001, p. 156). Thus a "counter-story-in-the-making" in SST has to concern itself with revising identity. Our responsibility in SST, when involved in co-authoring a counter-story, is to get on to a storyline involving self-redefinition that will resist and eventually replace a narrative that negatively defines one's identity to such an extent that they experience oppression.

Inviting a Counter-Story

A counter-story involves elevating a plot in juxtaposition to the problem plot. To invoke a counter-story I most often turn to externalizing conversations however re-authoring conversations can also be developed into counter-stories (see Ingamells, 2016). For me, externalizing conversations (White & Epston, 1990; White and Morgan, 2006; White, 2007) quickly provide the means to talk about experience in a way that invites the protagonist/antagonist relationship favourable to counter-storying. As discussed in Chapter 10, introducing the linguistic shift from adjectives used to describe oneself to nouns, introduces a play with language positioning internalized discourse (I am Depressed) as an external antagonist (Depression is stealing my hope). Invoking this relationship quickly sets the foundation for co-authoring a counter-story.

In the article *Brief narrative practice at the walk-in clinic: The rise of the counterstory* (Cooper, 2014) you were introduced to the story of Daniel[4] and the development of his counter-story. Let's revisit Daniel's story here to look more closely at this kind of conversation.

Daniel[5] was seen at a walk-in therapy clinic. He greeted me hesitantly, with eyes cast aside and a quiet "hey". A review of his pre-conversation paperwork offered only a hint about him. He had indicated very little other than he was "depressed" and wanted to "get help with his mental health". He had left the question, "When are things better, even a little bit?" blank, which is often a flag for me about the dominance of the Problem. The school social worker who accompanied this 14-year-old young person elaborated, noting how she was very worried because Daniel "is depressed" and has been "thinking about sui-cide". As an aside, when a service provider makes the time to bring someone to the walk-in, I am curious about their support. I wonder what it is that has them so concerned and also what it is they are valuing about the person to make time to connect them to service. To meet Daniel through the story of his worth and value, I asked permission to meet him through the social worker's eyes as she had known him for some time.

Daniel was open to this third-party introduction, so I began with the question, "What have you come to know and appreciate about this young person through the time you have had with him?" She described how Daniel had been in and out of foster care services, yet despite this, continues to be a caring person and remains especially close to his mother. She connects this to her sense that he "really cares about family". She goes on to note how he has always been kind and respectful to her, even when the situation has been disheartening and discouraging. She had brought him on this day out of her concern for him as *his* Depression seemed to be getting worse. She highlighted his diagnosis of Depression from early on in his life which Daniel confirmed with a nod of agreement and added that it's getting worse now to the point in which he doesn't want to do anything. He described how often he thinks to himself, "why even bother trying, nothing's going to get better". Hearing this, I am thinking to myself, is this a theme of helplessness or futility.

This is a good example of how despite efforts to facilitate a conversation with an initial focus on competency, the Problem can find a way in, taking up airtime to define a person. To reclaim our talk from It, I checked in with Daniel about what the staff had initially said to which he confirmed his value for family, how he doesn't give up on them, and he knows they are trying their best. He evi-dences this, sharing that he is now back living with his mother, and she is doing well. This is a circumstance that he is thankful for and notes it is a step towards how he wants things to be.

Listening for Plot and Counter-plot

As noted in Chapter 4, listening with a "brief narrative ear", in part, involves listening for the dominant plot and contradictions to that plot (White, 1995). In listening for plot, I am not listening solely for the problem and material outside the problem but rather, I take a zoomed-out vantage point, listening for the overarching theme or plot line to be countered. Plot reflects the theme given to events and the meaning made of the events of life. Eliciting a "counter-plot" and strengthening it through eliciting events, ideas, and thoughts that contradict the problem plot, provides a path not only to new or revised ways of proceeding but towards the consideration of a more preferred identity.

Problematic plot lines may reflect notions of incompetence (White, 1995), helplessness, futility, personal failure (White, 2002), and mistrust, to name a few. As the dominant plot is revealed, counter themes become available such as competence, purpose, perseverance, personal agency, protest, resistance, or testament, inviting a broader range of inquiry. The practice is to seek experiences that further inform these counter-themes. When experiences are brought into a counter-theme they find greater meaning, association, and simply make more sense.

The characterization of Daniel as Depressed seemed to shape an overarching theme of *helplessness* reflected in his statement "why bother trying". My concern was that he was rendered as powerless to affect what he was experiencing within that storyline. Daniel expressed a longing for things to be different in his life yet saw no way forward. Responding to the theme of helplessness, a counter-story needed to canvas a renewed sense that he could direct his life and a self-definition that would sponsor new options for proceeding in life. This involves a very different process than listening solely for contradictions to the problem of Depression. Contradictions void of a broader theme would have limited our conversation to times when he experienced less "depression" or was "not as depressed". The conversation would have centered around the concept of "Depression". Although those experiences are important, it's possible they would have lacked the meaning sufficient to resist the dominant narrative of helplessness.

Meeting the Protagonist

Externalizing conversations establish a protagonist/antagonist relationship between the person and the problem. At this point, as part of our general ethic of practice, I have taken time to meet our protagonist Daniel through stories of competence, away from the Problem,[6] and through the eyes of his social worker. As a micro counter-storying practice, this serves to reclaim the conversation from the Problem and foreground preferred identity stories. In these conversations, we are quickly acquainted with material that begins a rehabilitation of identity despite what the Problem would have people believe. What stood out for me was his care for family as evidenced in his unwavering love of his mother and enduring hope for a relationship with his father.

Meeting the Antagonist

I have also taken time with Daniel to have him introduce me to the Antagonist named Depression. Externalizing the problem provides a space for the recognition and naming of the problem as the Antagonist in contrast to positioning the person as the Protagonist. I meet the Antagonist through an exploration of the "relative influence of the Problem on the person"; Externalizing Conversations Map 1 (White & Epston, 1990). This invites a shift in the way the Protagonist perceives the world of the Antagonist making visible the Problem's oppression of the Protagonist.

White's externalizing conversations statement of position map one assisted Daniel to characterize and name the Problem of "Depression". He shared how *It* had him feeling down and drained of energy. He often experienced sadness, had trouble sleeping and thoughts about suicide. It struck me how Daniel's expression of his distress fit the stock plot characterization of the diagnosis of depression. When Depression was dominating him, small things felt big, and he couldn't clear his mind from the kind of thinking that he came to name "Discouraging Talk of a Crappy Day". That talk was often typified by statements such as "don't bother trying because you're just going to fail", "you're the reason your dad's not around", "you're useless", "you're a disappointment", "you can't do anything", and at its worst "maybe you should just kill yourself".[7]

To further the characterization of the Problem, I listed on paper these statements and invited reflection upon the list that included an exploration of the effects of these thoughts and the intentions of the externalized problem. Remember, lists can provide a useful take-away document for future reference. In these circumstances I simply fold a blank piece of paper in half. On one half I record the Problem talk and effects. On the contrasting side, I record the counter-knowledge, counter-voice and counter-steps people have taken. In counter-storying, lists quickly and visually juxtapose the voice and effects of the Problem with the counter-voice and intentions of the Person.

You have to listen closely for the counter-voice. It can be heard in statements such as, "I know that's just the Depression talking, it's not really me" or "*sometimes* I think it's no use[8]". These statements hint towards what the Protagonist knows outside of the Antagonists oppression. Other times, you can elicit this voice through further inquiry such as, "I imagine that you haven't always thought this way and that you know some things about yourself that this Depression has tried to hide from you or silence. Can you tell me about that?". Through this inquiry Daniel's counter-knowledge started to become visible.

Naming the Plot/Counterplot

As our single session conversation proceeds it becomes necessary to rough in together a name for the plot and counterplot. Naming in single session practice, as discussed in Chapter 6 and 7, is important to quickly develop a frame in which other initiatives and exceptions can be mapped, associated, and linked (Zimmerman & Dickerson 1996). Remember a stand-alone initiative is likely easily forgotten or discounted but several events linked together have greater endurance. In the same way I seek a name for the story-in-the-making, I seek a name for the counter-plot working with people to put words to what is counter to the problem story OR reflects their activities that fit with their preferences. These names often build from the contrasting list of the protagonist/antagonist characterization I have mentioned earlier. The names of counter-stories often involve movement metaphors such as the beginning of "life projects", "journeys", or "steps" (see Freedman & Combs, 2002, pp. 21–24.; White, 2004, pp. 44–57).

Understanding what Lindemann Nelson (2001) refers to as the "faces of oppression" assists with recognizing plot and counterplots and the naming process. If we hear Problems as marginalizing, exercising the "…unjust exclusion of people from participation in life" (p. 109), we are invited to canvas experiences informing a counter project of "reclaiming" domains of life. Hearing the "violence" of Problems as "…members live in fear of attacks that are motivated by nothing but the desire to humiliate, hurt or destroy them" (p. 111), compelling counter plots of "Self-care steps", "Survival", and "Steps for MY future" emerge especially in the face of problems such as bullying, problematic eating, or personal injury.

Returning to the story of Daniel, he had become "…supervised by the professional rather than supervised by the self" (p.110). The know-how and local wisdom of the protagonist and his family was discounted as the Problem had enforced a sense of "powerlessness". Universal science shaped who he was as he became "…represented by that science" (p.110). When we hear a Problems enforcement of "powerlessness", counter-story themes related to the revival of personal agency are negotiated such as "My breakup with depression", or "Being the boss of myself". These themes support a shift to Whites (2011) "second posture" ' in which "…people initiate action to diminish the influence of the problem and to pursue what they identified as important to them" (p. 30). Questions inviting naming may include:

- Okay so you have been blocked from living the life you want by the "wall of depression", what would you call this project you have started today in working to reclaim your life and future from Depression? A: "Taking Apart the Wall".
- When you look back at these developments what would you call this journey you have embarked on if you could give it a name?
- What would you call that? Is this like a "step for safety" or a "stand for safety" in a sense?
- Okay so if you connect all these initiatives together and were to give them a name that reflects the journey you're on, what would you call it? What might the title be? Answer: "Dismantling the Wall of Depression!"

Contextualizing Distress

Contextualizing distress invites important details to the foreground renewing meaning making. Contextualizing or contexting refers to the ways in which our questions foreground what people have been through, the context of their life. Contexting assists people to make sense of their experiences, placing them within a timeline and social and relational history. It assists with the linking of events and meanings made of those events. It is within the context of life that counter-story fragments can be found.

There is always context to people's experience of distress. If distress is de-contextualized, that is seemingly out of nowhere I send people back to their doctor to rule out physical contributions that show up as worry, sadness, moodiness, or aggression. Ailments such as celiac disease or gluten intolerance, diabetes, B12 deficiency, anemia, thyroid anomalies, and central auditory processing differences are useful to have ruled out. I tell families that we don't want to be six months in addressing mental health when there was an unidentified physical contribution. Over the years we have had many of these identified. For young children, these include pediatric autoimmune neuropsychiatric disorders associated with streptococcal infection (PANDAS) or behaviours related to acquired head injury.

Daniel had come to understand his distress as an aberration of his mind. I sought links between the context of his life and the description of Depression. He and his social worker shared that, as a young boy, he had been in and out of foster homes as his mother struggled with addiction. His father was frequently absent from his life, which had Daniel understanding himself as unwanted and unloved. With multiple school changes, his education was full of gaps contributing to the conclusion that he was stupid. It was in this contextualizing of experience that it came to light that Depression had come into his life in response to the widening gap between his life circumstances and the life he wanted for himself. He came to say that Depression was uninvited and like "a wall" surrounding him and limiting his world. He wasn't going to accept (It's) place in his life any longer. The context of his experiences provided extensive meaning making material to draw into the developing counter-story.

Further Developing the Protagonist/Antagonist Relationship

Attention to specifically fostering the protagonist/antagonist relationship assists to grow a compelling counter-story. This is a relationship in which our protagonist becomes increasingly centred in the storyline, opposing the named antagonist. Literary theory suggests a well-written protagonist is active. They know what they <u>want</u>, they know what is in their <u>way</u> and they know what they are going to <u>do</u> about it (Pace, 2014). Weaving these threads into the unfolding counter narrative serves to bring forward how protagonists act on the world, mustering their resolve while canvasing their determination to overcome the Problem.

1. Questions to Render the Protagonist as Active

These questions foreground how the Protagonist has been active despite the oppression of the Problem. This recognizes that people remain active in resistance to oppression. Our questions serve to elicit this activity as it is compelling and provides fertile ground for making more visible what is in the way and what can be done about it.

- In the face of those lies Depression was trying to have you believe, what did you do to carry on, to refuse to be completely persuaded by Its discouragement talk?
- As Depression clouded your view of the world how did you respond? Was the "shutting down" a way of protecting yourself from the harsh treatment in experiencing bullying?
- The Depression had you consider killing yourself, yet you refused. How did you hold on to the possibilities ahead for your life?

2. Questions to Make Visible what the Protagonist Wants

Questions that elicit what the Protagonist wants, serve to bring into further contrast the intentions of the Antagonist with the wishes of the Protagonist. I want to elicit the Protagonist's preference for one plot or the other. Becoming more richly acquainted with what they want, the protagonist's agenda becomes clearer and more within reach. With that agenda coming visible teamwork is invited as meaningful relations can play a part in the agenda or project.

- So, if you gave your life over to the Problem what kind of life would it want for you?
- Is that okay with you or do you have a picture of the life you want for yourself? What is it that you want more for yourself? How would you prefer things to be in your life?
- Do you prefer to be in charge of your own life or are you fine with Depression directing you?

3. Questions to Make Visible What Stands in the Protagonist's Way

These are questions that make the antagonist more visible and further implicated in the interference of the protagonist's life and preferences. The intention of these questions is to muster a revised attitude towards the antagonist. The attitude sought is one that is equal or exceeding that of the Problem (Freeman et al., 1997, p. 98).

- Is it my understanding then that this Problem stands defiantly in your way to more of the kind of life you want for yourself, like a wall?
- Given your up-close experience with this Problem what is your understanding about how it gets in your way of thinking good thoughts about yourself?
- This Problem has brought its tyranny into your life and continues to steal from you your fun and friendships. With what level of your own determination do you want to address "Its" next attempts to mess with your future?

Collecting Counter-Story Fragments

Drawing from past events, I elicit and document the fragments of stories outside the problem story. These could involve events, actions, intentions, hopes, and dreams that relate to the counter-story theme as well as counter thoughts/ feelings/actions that may be counterpoint to the problem. The idea is through collaboration with the family to bring those fragments into a collection related to the counter-story theme that begins the "rehabilitation of identity" (Lindeman Nelson, 2001), and sets the stage for the noticing and/or addition of future experiences congruent with the developing storyline.

With Daniel's assistance the scene was unfolding in which the external entity of Depression known as the antagonist in his life, had purpose and intention. He was clear that he wanted what he called "the Wall of Depression" taken apart. In response to inquiry seeking contradictions to the plot of *helplessness*, Daniel described a previous life in which he could do something to make himself happy. These experiences involved a counter voice of "encouragement" and experiences of directing his life more towards his wishes. He had friends and left the house more. He exercised an ability to clear his mind, work through what was going to happen, and use breathing to bring relief. He recalled times at school in which he told himself "I have to start working towards my goals and trying even if I know I might fail, I still need to do it". He explained this was a talk counter to "discouragement talk" and led him to greater success at school.

Daniel reflected on more recent developments such as his father's efforts to have a relationship with him. This had fostered a realization that his father's absence was not his fault or due to a problem with him as a son; an idea Depression would have had him believe. As if this realization provided an off-ramp to other counter developments, Daniel shared with some enthusiasm that his mother was doing good too; the way she used to be as she was around more and happier. These developments put into question the "self-blame" he had experienced for the adults' past actions. As these counter-story fragments were collected they became associated and linked under a theme beginning to counter helplessness while hinting at a revived identity storied as able and cared about. Although the counter-story at this time in the conversation may not be significant enough to dislodge the dominant narrative, the process has begun, and further practices will serve to stretch the story out into the real world.

Assisting the Endurance of the Counter-Story

While a freshly formed counter-story can be compelling, it too remains vulnerable to fading after a single session. As noted in Chapter 7, it's important to tend to the endurance of the story-in-the-making. Here too, we want to ask questions that set the stage for the noticing of events that grow the counter-story. This will serve to inoculate it against future assimilation by the Problem. Travelling within the Conversation Endurance Map, I was able to ask Daniel questions to discern what he would take with him from our conversation as a means to begin to rough in proposals for action in the real world. With Daniel these questions were explored following a short re-telling[9] of our conversation:

- Given what we have talked about today what idea would be useful to keep with you when you leave here or what might be something to try out as a next step?
- Suppose you were to continue dismantling the wall of depression when you leave here today, how would you specifically go about it? What will be the first thing you do when you leave here today that is guided by You rather than by the Depression?

Daniel experienced talking as useful and noted he needed to find someone he could talk to that was reliable and trustworthy. He identified a few people he had in mind, and he planned to approach them. He also thought Depression would want to keep him from doing the things he wanted to do so he decided he needed to find an activity; something to do that he enjoyed. We recorded these next steps on his conversation summary. Daniel was confident he could successfully take these steps to begin to dismantle the wall of Depression.

The second territory of the Conversation Endurance Map invites the protagonist into wild speculation about how the unfolding counter-story and proposals for action will shape their life after the conversation. I am inviting Daniel to re-contextualize the counter-story and situate the proposals for action into his everyday life. It's also a means to further expand the possibilities through the unfolding counter-story.

- Where will you try that out? When would be a good time to have that idea with you, when you need it the most?
- Suppose you do that what difference do you suppose that will make? What will it make possible?
- What will you come to know more about yourself that Depression had tried to blind you and others from?

Together, we loitered in a conversation about how the person he would talk to might respond and the difference that would make to Daniel. He imagined having someone to talk to would help him to keep his mind out of the "discouragement" and more focused on his "reassurance talk". Talking and having an activity would help him to know he was "growing", and the "wall of Depression" was coming down. In place of the wall would be an "open path" forward.

Thirdly, enduring counter-stories must be widely circulated and witnessed to counter and eventually displace the problem story. I invited Daniel to audience his story, asking him to think about and highlight who it may be important to share this counter narrative with, how might he share it, and how might those named respond?[10]

- Who would it be important to share this story with when you leave here?
- How might they respond knowing about these developments?
- How will this begin to shift how they have come to know you?

Daniel discussed sharing the emerging story with his mother and the social worker who had earlier left the room to let Daniel have his privacy. He noted those folks would help him "take apart the wall of Depression".

As part of counter-storying too, I invite people to co-develop "take-away documents" archiving the counter-story that can be shared and consulted further as needed. Although Daniel had identified some clear next steps to begin to take apart the wall of Depression, I remained concerned that the Problem-story would be difficult to dislodge given the influence of diagnosis, and the context of Daniels' life in which he found school difficult. To further extend the emerging counter-story, Daniel was invited to co-craft the following letter addressed to Depression sharing his new understandings and the change in relationship with Depression that was unfolding.[11]

Dear Depression,

I have some things you need to know. I'm taking apart the wall and you probably won't like that. You have been making me feel really really bad about myself and life in general. You try to convince me to not even try to do my schoolwork or do the things I need to do because you want me to think I'm setting myself up for failure. Yes, I'm worried about failing BUT I know I have to try and take chances in order to do things to succeed. Failing is part of how to learn in life! You try to hide hope from me and make me think there is only darkness for my future. I've had enough of your constant drag down. Now, here's even harder news for you.

I have a clear vision of myself and the kind of life I want to build. I am a nice person and I have strength to overcome many things. I'm good at English and art. But there is more. There are things that are really important to me such as being the first in my family to complete high school, my family, my friends, running my own life, being who I am. I will keep strong with these ideas and of how I want to live my life.

I understand that you came into my life during hard times. BUT now things are better, even though you still drag me down. I'm not who I used to be or who you want me to be. I am taking old weight off of my shoulders like figuring out that it's not my fault that my dad was in and out of my life so many times. He owns that not me. I'm not that violent kid I used to be. My mom has made changes and I have too. So, things are going to start changing with you as well. You are no longer something I keep bottled up and hidden. You are now out in the open and being dealt with. You may not like that but it's what I want. I have people I trust and can now talk to about you. I'm getting stronger and stronger every day to deal with this. Soon you'll be gone and I won't be worrying about you. Then I can live my life the way I want.

So depression, this is your notice to pack your stress and bad things that have me angry and sad to take them with you. This may take a while but it's going to happen whether you like it or not.

Throughout the letter the theme of exercising personal agency; "the conduct of action under the sway of intentional states" (Bruner 1990, p 9.) counters the original problem dominating theme of helplessness. The crafting of the letter itself is acting upon the Problem, directing his life with intention towards how he wants it to be. As part of the Conversation Endurance Map, I asked Daniel where it would be useful to keep the letter and when and how often would it be useful to read the letter should Depression try to wall him in. He speculated that it would be important to read this letter to himself three times a day or should he start to "feel down". We note that on his conversation summary. He thought he would share this with his mother and the school social worker who had brought him on this day. Others have shared their letters more widely, posted them on Facebook or circulated copies to the significant people in their life.

Lastly, assuming the resistance of the antagonist, I engage people in speculation about what might try to get in the way of preferred developments, cause setbacks or invite the re-emergence of the problem. Once identified, counter plans can be developed.

- When you take these steps, how might the Problem try to discourage you or re-establish the hold on your life it had for so long?
- If that was to happen, how will you counter it? What actions will you take?
- What will you say to yourself or remind yourself about to remain on this path?

Daniel identified that returning to school could be difficult as it was a place in which he experienced failure and bullying. He supposed, in that setting, it would be much harder to dismantle the wall of Depression. He speculated that it would be useful to have more "talks" like the one we had that day.[12]

Closing

This chapter has shared practices for the development of counter-stories through externalizing practice in brief narrative single session therapy. Counter-stories, being a specific kind of story, involve the juxtaposition of counter plot to the problem plot and set out to rehabilitate a compromised identity. Gathering counter-story fragments, linking them into a counter-plot and bringing into question the things a dominant story can try to claim about a person can help open the way to new possibilities. Although in the time constrained context of therapeutic walk-in clinic conversations counter-stories are vulnerable to eclipse by the problem narrative, there are ways to inoculate it and assist it to further thicken well after the initial face to face contact.

Notes

1 Erving Goffman, (1963) used the term "spoiled identity" discussing circumstances when identity has gone wrong or there is an ascription of stigma from notions of identity. I find this term very useful framing the effects of the dominant discourse of pathology and its effects on people.

2 What I refer to as dominant story Lindemann Nelson commonly refers to as master narrative. Language evolves and as such I prefer to use the term "dominant" as the word "master", for some, conjures images of plantation slavery. I am cognizant that where I live and work there is a history of slavery and on-going colonialism. The legacy of this oppression continues today evidenced as we continue to work towards racial justice, equity, liberation, and community.

3 Lindemann Nelson contends that…[dominant] …narratives are widely circulated stories in cultures that, "…serve as summaries of socially shared understandings" (p. 6). They "… are often archetypal, consisting of stock plots and readily recognizable character types…[and] … ignore or underplay details and complexity" (p.6.). As such, [dominant] narratives are influential and oppressive in constricting meaning making and serving as justifications for people's actions. Consequently, they are resistant to change and difficult to dislodge.

4 The name Daniel is an alias and details have been modified to ensure privacy.

5 Parts of this chapter have been previously shared in the article: Cooper, S. Brief narrative practice at the walk-in clinic: The rise of the counterstory [online]. *International Journal of Narrative Therapy & Community Work*, No. 2, 2014: [23–30] and are reprinted here with permission.

6 Away from the Problem conversations are in harmony with David Epston's Wonderfulness enquiries, learning about what people have to put up against the Problem whatever that might be.

7 This expression may invite the reader to experience concern for Daniel's safety. Although walk-in clinic therapy is most often a single session, safety is a priority. Should safety remain a concern following any conversation steps are initiated to co-identify and assemble a circle of care to shore up safety in the face of distress. With respect to Daniel, he had a long history of resisting killing himself that was foregrounded in our conversation. He identified several people in his circle of care including the school social worker who he saw often. Further he was acquainted with and agreeable to using the community 24-hour child and youth crisis phone service should distress try to take his future possibilities from him. Although we may hear these kinds of expressions often at the walk-in clinic, with the development of a compelling counter-story, the Problem may have far less influence by the end of a single session. When the person is no longer viewed as the problem several alternative means to address the problem come more available bringing greater safety for proceeding in life.

8 The word "sometimes" hints that there are other times when they are thinking differently. Those contrasting thoughts can be canvased and added to the counter-voice.

9 It's important to remember this specific re-telling shared as we near the end of our conversation is more than a recounting of events. It is storied and derived from the exact words used in the conversation, juxtaposing the problem story and counter-story, highlighting a turning point in which the Protagonist takes centre stage in the journey.

10 White and Epston, 1990, have shaped this category of inquiry for me in their discussion of "unique circulation questions". They note how "the scope of alternative stories can be further extended through the introduction of questions that invite persons to identify and recruit an audience to the performance of new meanings in their life" (p. 41).

11 It is not uncommon for people to take an impassioned adversarial posture towards the Problem as the counter-story unfolds. However, the intention is not to vilify the antagonist recognizing some Problems come into people's lives for very important

reasons and as meaningful responses to the context of their life. Counter-story development reflects a shift in relation to the antagonist, rendering the Problem less dominating of the person while no longer defining their identity. In these conversations and in the take-away documents there is opportunity to acknowledge the importance of the problem at one time in the protagonists' life and to recognize the wish or intention to modify the relationship. There are times as well when it is fitting to thank the antagonist for assisting the protagonist through hard times yet notifying it that it will no longer define the person or hold them back from what they want different in their life.

12 At the time of this conversation Daniel was on wait for a short term eight session therapy. Approximately a month following his walk-in conversation Daniel participated in that short-term service model and continued to thicken the counter-story begun at the walk-in clinic. That service also assisted to address the effects of poverty and bullying on Daniel's life. Although he has continued to have ups and downs in his life for the year following, he had not had to use crisis services, had resumed full time classes at school and was not involved in therapy services.

References

Bruner, E. M. (1986). Experience and its expressions. In V. W. Turner & E. M. Bruner (Eds.), *The anthropology of experience* (pp. 3–30). University of Illinois Press.

Cooper, S. (2014). Brief narrative practice at the walk-in clinic: The rise of the counterstory [online]. *International Journal of Narrative Therapy and Community Work,* 2: 23–30.

Freedman, J. & Combs, G. (2002). *Narrative therapy with couples… and a whole lot more! A collection of papers, essays and exercises.* Adelaide: Dulwich Centre Publications.

Freeman, J., Epston, D. & Lobovits, D. (1997). *Playful approaches to serious problems: Narrative therapy with children and their families.* New York: W.W. Norton.

Goffman, E. (1963). *Stigma: Notes on the management of spoiled identity.* Engelwood Cliffs, NJ: Prentice Hall.

Ingamells, K. (2016). Learning how to counter-story in narrative therapy (With David Epston and Wilbur the Warrior). *Journal of Systemic Therapies. 35:* 58–71. 10.1521/jsyt.2016.35.4.58.

Lindemann, N. H. (2001). *Damaged identities, narrative repair.* New York: Cornell University Press.

Pace, B. (2014). 4 Steps to creating a truly active protagonist retrieved Jan 20, 2014 from www.scripteach.com/?page_id=667

White, M. (1995). *Re-authoring lives: Interviews & essays.* Adelaide, Australia: Dulwich Centre Publications.

White, M. (2002). Addressing personal failure. *The International Journal of Narrative Therapy and Community Work,* 3.

White, M. (2004). Working with people who are suffering the consequences of multiple trauma: A narrative perspective. *International Journal of Narrative Therapy and Community Work,* (1), 45–76. Reprinted in D. Denborough, (Ed.). (2006). *Trauma: Narrative responses to traumatic experience* (pp. 25–85). Adelaide, Australia: Dulwich Centre Publications.

White, M. (2007). *Maps of narrative practice*. New York: W.W. Norton.

White, M. (2011). *Narrative practice: Continuing the conversations*. W.W. Norton, New York.

White, M. & Epston, D. (1990). *Narrative means to therapeutic ends*. New York: W.W. Norton.

White, M. & Morgan A. (2006). *Narrative therapy with children and their families*. Adelaide, Australia: Dulwich Centre Publications.

Zimmerman, J. & Dickerson, V. (1996). *If problems talked: Narrative therapy in action*. New York: Guilford Press.

Chapter 12

Addressing the Effects of Trauma in a Single Session

In this chapter, I will share how narrative practice assists in addressing the effects of trauma in single session encounters. For many, the idea of discussing what is considered trauma within a single session can be challenging. Fortunately, there are many narrative influenced examples in the literature demonstrating time constrained narrative approaches to trauma themed conversations and we can take inspiration from these. They hint at what is possible. Strong and Flynn (2000) co-author an account of a single narrative therapy conversation with a man who had witnessed the shooting of hundreds of North Korean prisoners of war at Camp Koji Do. He related his distress to that incident. Perdomo (2017) shares creative documenting in single session therapy to move meaning from a context of trauma and post-traumatic stress disorder to one of abilities. Batrouney (2019), working single session telephone counselling, shares many uses of narrative practice with women who have experienced sexual violence. Similarly, Lumsden (2020) shares accounts of a narrative approach used at a domestic violence hotline in Japan. These examples offer what might be possible if we, as therapist, stay open to the idea that a conversation, when relevant and skillfully shared, can make a difference regardless of time constraint.

Sometimes the pre-session paperwork will outline that people have come specifically to talk about what they have been through. Other times, the conversation may take a turn and a "trauma story"[1] is shared without forewarning. In these moments it's useful for the therapist to have ideas about how to navigate the conversation in a way that is not only useful in meeting what the participant wanted out of the time but is also safe enough. White (2006) emphasizes our responsibility as caretakers in these conversations, asking:

- How do we have conversations in which people do not re-experience distress of the past?
- How do we have conversations that assist people not to get stuck in the immediacy of their experience as they re-tell events of their lives?
- How do we best tend to psychological and emotional safety of the people in these conversations?

DOI: 10.4324/9781003431688-13

Responding to the questions and in order to lay a path of conversational options, let's first look at the discourse of trauma and how widely circulated ideas about trauma tends to shape the therapy and ideas about what is possible or not.

Noticing the Discourse of Trauma

The concept of "trauma" itself is not benign. It has come to mean many things to many people, spanning the fields of psychology, psychiatry, neurobiology, and medicine. It has become an industry on its own and, as such, a discourse shaping therapeutic conversations in profound ways. "Discourses are the underlying beliefs that structure and guide people's thoughts, feelings, and actions in a given culture" (Beaudoin, M-N, 2004, p. 510).

White (2003) makes visible the discourse of trauma, linking the word to "naturalistic" accounts of pain and distress. He notes how emotional pain, distress, and suffering from the experience of trauma are constructed in Western culture similar to physical injury. Trauma, understood as an internal wound and compressed emotions, shapes a healing project described through cathartic metaphors of getting things out, releasing emotion, working through the events, over a great deal of time. He highlights how these ideas have shaped therapy, prioritizing practices that have people revisit and recount traumatic events to work through them. He expresses concern about how this practice risks re-traumatizing people.

Reynolds (2020) too, invites scrutiny of the modern conceptualization of trauma and trauma work. Through a critical analysis, she makes visible how trauma as a medicalized term with a focus on personal deficiencies has consequences for the practice of therapy. The effects of trauma, when medicalized and located within people, risks narrowing the conversation to symptom surveillance, assessment, and prescription, while concealing structural oppression and violence.

Clark (2016), subjecting the dominant discourses of trauma to a decolonizing lens notes how "Trauma discourse has become part of the mainstream narrative in Indigenous and non-Indigenous communities, globally and locally" (p. 4). She outlines how dominate trauma discourse colludes with ongoing colonization, shaping services that "…further colonize and pathologize Indigenous children and youths' health and their bodies" (p. 3). This has social and political implications. As SST is not exempt from replicating these politics, ongoing attention to relational ethics is called for.

In becoming aware of the discourse of trauma and associated therapeutic practices, we are able to reflect on how that discourse shapes what is thought to be possible or not in time constrained conversations. I want to emphasize that, from my experience, staying open to what might be possible in these conversations is very important. Further, growing a diverse repertoire of questions informed by the territories of curiosity discussed in Chapter 4, equips you to receive the story of distress differently, as contextual, with broader connections and associations than that of a biomedical lens. Again, we can only hear and see what we train ourselves to hear and see. How might you teach yourself to hear beyond the story arc of the dominant discourses of trauma? Separating from the discourse of trauma and medicalized distress serves to open new paths to possibility in these conversations.

Trauma as Un-Storied Events

In contrast to naturalistic and medicalized definitions of trauma and with story (events linked through time according to a theme) as a guiding framework, we are positioned to work with meaning making regarding people's experience of traumatic events. White (2003) explains the concept of trauma as representing people's experience of an event(s) that is irreconcilable with "themes about life that are cherished" and irreconcilable with "preferred accounts of one's identity". As such, we can understand traumatic events as un-storied or satellite to the many preferred storylines of people's lives.

As un-storied events, they are afloat, not tethered within the temporal flow like events situated within a storyline with a beginning and ending. When satellite and unanchored by storied meaning, people are vulnerable to reliving them at unanticipated times and in unforeseen ways. They can intrude into everyday life sparked and cued by a variety of everyday circumstances such as smells, sounds, tones, or phrases.

White (2005) speaks about the memories of these events as dis-associated memories in that they cannot be associated (linked or connected into chains of association) with those memories that encompass all the different storylines of people's lives. They are not associated with the memory of preferred events or stories of preferred identity. This experience is often reflected in people's descriptions of life as "feeling not themselves", "floating through life", "without substance", "numb", "in a dream like state", "having lost their way" or "as though observing life rather than living it". As a result, people draw or are ascribed very negative conclusions about themselves, their lives, and relationships. They may come to know themselves as broken, vulnerable or disordered.

Given this, we approach all conversations thinking about what storying can we take part in together that honours what people have been through yet proves useful in addressing what they come for. How can we talk in ways that are safe and assist people to make sense of their distress in a way that fits with their preferred view of themselves, relationships, and life in general? How can we assist the emerging story-in-the-making to then ripple out and be there for them when needed? For this project, it helps to distinguish between the story of pain and the story of possibility.

The First Story

As people share about traumatic experiences and the aftermath, the content is often dominated by talking about what they have been through and descriptions of the effects of the trauma. These accounts have people drawing negative identity conclusions about themselves, "this happened and ever since I have been...". These negative identity stories may include themes of personal failure, sense of helplessness, futility of life, self-blame, and shame. We can understand this account as the first story (White, 2004) related to the event(s).

The first story is about what they have been through, endured, and the effects of those circumstances. Very often, this is the story that people come to talk about. It is important to tend to the first story, and honour what people have been through should they want to share about it. However, it is equally important in a single session to foreground more preferred meanings. I do not want to dwell in the first story or have people re-experience the past in its telling. However, we do need to receive enough about this story to learn about peoples' responses. To structure safety, I may let them know I might interrupt periodically to elicit material outside the story of distress. There is always material to draw from outside the first story.

Second Story Development

While it is important to hear and honour the first story should someone want to share it, in time constrained conversations it becomes vital to also hear and expand the entry points that will provide paths to the story-in-the-making. Often eclipsed by the first story are events and intentional actions that go unnoticed and consequently un-storied. These are people's responses and resistance to the circumstance. White (2004) orients us to this material, noting, "No one is a passive recipient of trauma. People always take steps to try to prevent the trauma, and, even if preventing the trauma is clearly impossible, they take steps to try to modify it in some small way or to modify its effects on their lives, or they take steps in efforts to preserve what is precious to them" (p. 47).

Inquiring about people's responses and resistance to oppression (Reynolds, 2020), and what these actions are founded on in relation to values, beliefs, and intentions for life, provides the material for what White (2004) has referred to as the "second story". The first/second story dichotomy is used to contrast the story of harm and subsequent effects to the story of responses and the values responses are connected to. He has also called the second story the subordinate story, as it is often composed of experience rendered less significant or invisible in the world of popular trauma discourse.

In brief narrative conversations, I am vitally interested in the development of the second story-in-the-making. It involves first identifying ways people have responded to what they were subjected to. Second, we link those responses to what they reflect about what is important to people, such as values or beliefs. Third, we link response to certain knowledge and skills and trace the history of all this material linking to family, community, culture. Finally, we explore how the emerging second story can make a difference to them in the real world.

The second story is also a story of revised identity. Within this story-in-the-making, people come to know themselves in ways that counter or, in the least, contest what the first story would have them believe about themselves and their future. Second story development begins the rehabilitation of identity, so to speak, as counter claims emerge that are more preferred.

A Map for Navigating Trauma Conversations in SST

Many derivative narrative-informed conversation maps have been crafted to guide conversations with those suffering the effects of trauma (White, 2005; Beaudoin, 2005; Yuen, 2007, 2009, 2019). These maps come to life within specific contexts and durations of service. The context of a brief narrative single session conversation is unique in that you have no prior relationship with the participant and may not see them again to repair mishaps. Within the remainder of this chapter, I will share a map to address the effects of trauma relevant to brief narrative single session therapy. I will begin by describing some key processes including structuring safety, and double listening before outlining the four levels of inquiry that contribute to second story development.

Structuring Safety

As a key process, structuring safety (Richardson & Reynolds, 2014) emphasizes the important responsibilities we hold for how we facilitate conversations with people suffering from the effects of trauma. As discussed in Chapter 5, phase one directs attention to how we convene these gatherings. Being clear about the process to come, asking permission to ask our questions, and letting people know they do not have to answer any questions we ask, are all acts to structure safety. In practice, as we begin, I note that I tend to ask a lot of question and if I ask a question that I don't have business asking or that is not useful, I invite the person to let me know. I may also note that at any time I sense that a question is too bothersome, I will check in with them and may alter course as well. In this way, I am alerting them to my process, as well as offering a say in how we proceed as co-travellers on the conversational journey.

Throughout the conversation, I also ask permission to ask questions about specific topics. I do not assume I have permission to do so because, as Tom Anderson (in Malinen et al., 2012) has said, our questions, at times, can be experienced as punches. Further, I will note why I am asking what I am asking to embrace transparency. I may say:

I'm wondering if it would be okay if I asked more about what you went through. I won't ask about what happened, but rather I am curious about how you responded. The reason I am curious about that is because no one is a passive recipient of abuse. People are always responding, and I am wondering about how you responded and if this leads us to ideas about your skills, and what is important to you. Would it be okay if I asked a few questions about this? Again, if a question is bothersome, please let me know and we'll alter course.

After discussing a safe enough context in which to have our conversation, I then concern myself with what story making is taking place in our time together. It is at this point that we separate from the modern concept of trauma to embrace distress as expressions of meaning, as actions founded on values and intentions for life, and as acts of resistance to what they have been through.

Understanding people's expressions in this way opens options for meaning making. I am listening for and curious about the second story, seeking to co-author stories that foster personal agency, rehabilitate identity, and foreground intentions for life. These are stories of hope and possibility that not only honuor what people have been through but seed what still might be that fits with a preferred future. To access this information, once again, we listen in a specific way.

Double Listen to the Expression of Distress

Another key process involves the skill of double listening for what is implied as explored in Chapter 4. Double listening means we are listening for two stories simultaneously. This involves receiving the first story while intentionally listening for what is implied in the expression of complaint. We listen for what people have been through and what their distress teaches about what they are separating from and wishing to move towards.

As the senior partner,[2] I may periodically interrupt, asking a question that points towards an opening for the second story, but being careful that this inquiry is not experienced as silencing. In receiving the first story it can help to remember that every expression is an action. An expression about the effects of trauma speaks to people's wish to be free of the distress, implying they have a picture of the preferred life they seek. This understanding assists us to resist getting mired solely in the first story.

Again, while it is important to hear what people wish to share about the first story, I simultaneously listen for and inquire about material to inform the second story. Specifically, with second story development in mind, I am listening for hints as to the person's responses to the trauma at the time and/or ongoing. With "responses" as a focus of this species of listening, what is understood as symptoms of pathology can be understood as responses to trauma.

Allan Wade, family therapist and researcher, and colleagues have developed a response-based approach to address the effects of violence. Wades work, in harmony with my brief narrative approach, has been a very useful resource, expanding what's possible in these conversations. According to Wade (1997) a response includes:

> Any mental or behavioral act through which a person attempts to expose, withstand, repel, stop, prevent, abstain from, strive against, impede, refuse to comply with, or oppose any form of violence or oppression (including any type of disrespect), or the conditions that make such acts possible, may be understood as a form of resistance.
>
> (p. 25)

Yuen (2007, 2019) highlights many kinds of responses she has learned from children experiencing trauma as she advocates for focusing on acts of resistance, protest, refusals to be silent or complicit, places of safety and other skills of living. Todd and Wade (2004) note how, "Emotional pain in response to violence signifies and registers a protest in that it shows that the victim is refusing to be contented, relaxed, and comfortable with abuse" (p. 152). Denborough (2008) has crafted a checklist of signs of social and psychological resistance to violence which presents a very practical way to elicit entry points to the second story. These folks have helped shape my listening.

Within the stories of those who have consulted to me, I have heard many diverse responses and hints at what these responses have been founded on. For example:

- Streaming tears have been the expression of a longing for safe and inclusive relationships.
- Sneaking and hiding has been a means to preserve safety in unsafe moments.
- Lying skills have been protective, as a means to lessen frequent assault.
- Freezing in stoic silence has been a way to disarm abuse.
- Not caring about what has happened has been a way to shield oneself from ongoing emotional pain and to escape hurt.
- Memory difficulties or stating "I don't know" can be understood as a protective practice allowing them not to revisit difficult experiences.
- Seeing figures that others don't is a refusal to be okay with trespass.
- Running away can serve as a means to escape to more preferred places and relations.
- Covering one's ears to quiet what is scary and/or demeaning and breaching values of respect and dignity.
- Protecting siblings or a parent as founded on the value of family and safety.
- Yelling or trying to negotiate as means of protest.

- Experiencing despair as tribute to how much someone values trust when it has been betrayed.
- Embracing fear as to never be caught off guard or be hurt again.
- Grieving as a way of honouring someone who has been lost and the intensity of that grief as a tribute to how important they were.
- Lying about or overly exaggerating positive stories about oneself as a means to say "please like me".
- Becoming overly skilled at reading the room for safety and risk as a means of preserving safety.

As we enter conversations about responses, we are mentored in the actions people have taken and the skills and knowledge they involve. We hear a range of responses that may register as acts of protest, protection, taking a stand for important beliefs and values, or refusals to be complicit with what has happened. These actions do not come out of nowhere but result from a connection to important values held which people, young or old, continue to try to stay connected to.

Transitioning to a Second Story

Movement into the second story involves a balance between honouring what people have been through and canvasing material for second story development. At times, people will describe their responses to trauma events as evidence of illness and disorder. Those expressions as Wade (1997) points out can often be heard as responses to what people have been through opening the way to an often-novel conversation. There are four levels of inquiry I try to progress through. Each level provides material to inform a second story, building in complexity moving through the middle phase of our conversation.

Level 1: Characterize the Response

The first level of the map involves characterizing the ways in which the person responded to what they have been through and co-developing a name for those responses. Answers may involve micro and macro responses such as what they did in the moment of the event and what they have been experiencing since. For instance, a child had been brought to walk-in following the family house burning down. They were struggling to attend school, not wanting to leave their parents' side. We came to learn that on the morning of the fire the child knew to exit the house and await family outside. They had "talked" themselves through the very "scary" event, telling themselves to get out of the house, leave their toys, and stay low like they had learned at school. These micro-responses came to be known as "quick thinking skills".

We also wondered together if "not wanting to be away from mom and dad" was a response of some kind and what kind of response might it be. This macro-response came to be understood and named as the "act of caring", and a way to ensure "family was safe". This new understanding was in contrast to the idea that the child was experiencing an emerging anxiety disorder. The revised understanding set a path for a very different kind of conversation.

So, level one of the map involves learning about and co-developing a name for the responses to what they have been through. To begin this conversation, we ask openly and directly about what people did or are doing since.

Ask Directly About Responses

Very often responses go unnoticed, and thus un-storied in a meaningful way. Through our inquiry we are eliciting responses and bringing them to the fore-ground into second story development. This involves direct inquiry about people's responses to what they have experienced and their ongoing responses (Yuen, 2019 p.127; Wade, 2007 p. 10). Together, we speculate about how the event(s) was handled. This line of questioning facilitates the experience of personal agency moving away from an effects-centric recall of their experience to a response-based conversation (Wade, 1997). We are locating sites of resistance to what has happened.

- How did you respond?
- What did you do?
- Given what you were going though, how did you handle it?
- Were there places you went to seeking safety or respite?
- Were their relationships you turned to for comfort, safety, or help?
- Were there people, toys, or pets you turned to?
- What did you think to yourself that helped to get through that bringing safety or comfort?

People have described many macro and micro responses. One young man shared with me how he used to urinate in his father's shampoo bottles as a means to protest his mistreatment in a way that went undetected and thus didn't make his situation worse. He had crafted ways of mocking his father where his father could not tell he was being mocked. Along with some expert skills at sneaking food, these responses helped him to get though the situation and register a protest to mistreatment. He noted reflecting on these acts of "standing up" to mistreatment, was very useful helping him to know even as a young child he knew what he experienced wasn't okay and he had done the best he could to protest.

Invite the Naming of the Response(s)

Naming the response assists it to become visible and taken up into broader themes linked to important intentions for life.

- What kind of response would you say that was?
- Would you say it was a protest of sorts, a way of refusing to be complicit?
- Was it protective in some way or taking a stand of some kind?
- What might you have been standing for and against?
- What if we thought of this numbness as a response to what you had been through? What kind of response might it be? Is it protective in some way?
- You said that ever since you've been feeling off and not yourself. What if we think about this feeling off and not yourself as a response to what you have been through, what kind of response might it be? Is it perhaps a way of saying you won't be silent about what happened?

As broader themes emerge fitting with intentions for life and connected to held values and beliefs, the second story-in-the-making begins to take shape.

Level 2: Linking

As every expression is plural, an expression of distress is not only an action towards preferred circumstances but also reflective of what matters to people. It reflects what is important to them and what they believe in. Listening for what's implied in the expression of complaint provides clues to what that might be. This material is foreground in second story development. I ask questions that assist people to link their actions to values, beliefs, intentions, and hopes for life.

Ask About What Matters to People

- Do you think the upset or distress relates to certain important values or beliefs that were trespassed in some way?
- Can you tell me a bit more about these values or beliefs?

  - Has that always been important to you?
  - Where else does that value show up in your life?

- If we think of Depression as a response to what has happened, what would you say it suggests about what you are not okay with that has gone on?
- What is it about what happened that doesn't sit right with you?
- What's your picture of how people should be treated in relationships?

Answers to these questions foreground how people value safety in relationships or safety in general. They make visible people's ideas about how life should be, including ideas such as peaceful, with kindness, respect, and inclusion. At times, connections can be made between how "what people went through" elevated these values and beliefs in their life and how they show up in the present. People seek justice, have committed to helping others, or express moral codes or pledges not to act how others have acted towards them.

Link to Their Knowledge and Skills

All responses are connected to certain knowledge and skills people employ known or unknown to them. Asking questions to elicit the knowledge and skills people have employed assist to language into existence their know-how and it's connect to their ability to take action.

- How did you know to do that?
- How did you decide to do that?
- How is it you managed to endure that for so long?
- What kind of skill/ability would you call that, self-care, protective, survival, an imagination skill, quick thinking, caring for others, lessening the circumstances skills?

People employ a broad range of skills in the face of hardship and answers to these questions are diverse and contextual. You may learn how someone has turned to their imagination to endure or how it made a difference to become an expert at reading the room to know when to get out. Still, others tap into their creativity, skills of focus or concentration, distraction, humour or acting to preserve their dignity and navigate trespass.

Level 3: Social and Relational Influence

Knowledge, skills, and what matters to people are grown and shaped in a social and relational process. We learn and are influenced through our interactions with family, friends, community, and cultural ethos. To infuse significance, we can invite people to link this material to their genealogy (Marsten et al., 2016) or as David Epston has said, to their hereditary lines of meaningful relationships in family, community, or culture. This is the act of populating the story-in-the-making by tracing what matters to people and learned skills back to relationships and other peripheral sources that have contributed to the value, belief, knowledge, skills.

Discover Hereditary Lines of Those Values, Beliefs, Knowledge and Skills

- Who introduced you to that belief/skill? Where did you learn that?
- What would they say if they knew you hold that belief still?
- Where did their knowledge come from?
- Who helped out even a bit?
- What did they do that you appreciate?
- Do they share some of the same beliefs and values as you?
- Is that approach to all living beings and relationships connected to your culture in some way?

Exploring these connections often presents the opportunity to navigate with the re-membering conversations map (White, 1997) to draw further connections through the dimensions of time and relationship.[3] For instance, a young boy brought for a single session consultation by his mother sought help to address the boy's experience of great sadness that was increasingly interfering with his everyday life for going on two years. His father had suffered a heart attack when the two were alone vacationing at an isolated cabin in the forest. Despite this, the boy knew to navigate the wilderness to bring back help. Unfortunately, his father had passed away. I came to learn how proud his father would have been to witness his son use his "survival skills" that he had taught him. They speculated how he would have been proud of his son and, in his last few hours, come to know he had done a good job as a dad evidenced by witnessing his son's bravery and skills in action. Reflecting upon this, the boy thought this idea that his dad would have known how good of a job he had done as a dad by witnessing his son's actions would be good to keep with him after the session. He noted how he hadn't realized this and that it would bring him some happiness to go along with the sadness when he misses his father.

Inquire About Revised Identity

These conversations are identity projects assisting people to come to know themselves in more preferred ways, countering the single story of the effects of trauma. Navigating the landscape of identity, we can invite people to speculate what the emerging second story suggests about them and who they are becoming.

- Given this discussion, what are you coming to know about yourself that is useful to you?

- What is it you are learning about yourself and what is possible for you as we have talked about this?
- Looking through your now 25-year-old eyes, what does it say about that younger you who responded refusing to be okay with what was happening?

I have heard many meaningful answers to this category of inquiry. People have described coming to know they were not a failure in the moment of trespass, but rather were acting in ways to preserve their life with intention to live a full life. Others, looking back at their younger selves and how they had navigated the horrors of life, had thought they were "courageous", "way smart for their age", "clever", or "strong". I've heard time and again people say how heart-warming it was to know that they held their values from a young age and what they went through had not been able to extinguish those values as they live into them still. Whereas the first story often paints people as docile, broken, and devaluing themselves, the second story-in-the-making begins to rehabilitate identity assisting people to know their competence, restored sense of personal agency and possibility.

Level 4: Re-Contextualize

This level of inquiry transitions to phase three of our brief narrative conversation in which we seek to assist people to contextualize what we have discussed back into everyday life. It is a time to discern next steps and set the stage for noticing future information that fits with the story-in-the-making. It involves the use of speculation on the landscape of action and the landscape of identity about how the "response-informed story-in-the-making" will ripple out into everyday life.

Contextualize the Second Story

Many people may be already making contributions to the world in harmony with what is important to them. However, we can ask about ways to keep this conversation with them and where it might show up in their life in useful ways. The phrasing is presuppositional, understanding that the conversation will ripple out into everyday life and make a useful difference.

- What was it like to have this conversation?
- How will what you are learning about yourself here today influence your life when you leave?
- Where else do you use those responses? What do they make possible for you? What does it suggest about the kind of world you are trying to shape?
- How do you continue to honour them?
- What difference will it make knowing trauma hasn't been able to take your beliefs and that you have been responding?

- What ideas are you having about how to continue on from here?
- Who else would it be important to involve?

Replies to these questions highlight emerging ideas and possible next steps people are considering. I hear answers such as, "It helps me to know I'm not crazy" to which I might follow up with "So instead of crazy, what are you knowing differently about yourself". They may say something like, "I did the best I could" or "What happened hasn't been able to steal what's important to me and in fact has only made it stronger". Receiving these answers provides opportunity to invite speculation about how this will shape life. I may say, "Suppose you were to keep that idea with you when you need it, what will it help you to do".

One participant described an image that had come to them as we talked of them and their child holding hands and walking along a favourite path. It was a safe and peaceful image and represented walking away from the trauma. They supposed it would be an important image to keep with them when they left and to revisit, especially during the times trauma tries to take them back in time to re-experience what they had endured. We detailed this image, ways to revisit it when needed, and the difference that would make in the future. While we weren't naive to more struggles ahead, the emerging second story about how this person could influence their distress provided hope and set the stage for a broader journey of continued growth.

While this chapter outlines a narrative therapy informed map for addressing the effects of trauma in single session therapy, I want to stress that this map is one of many that can assist in meaning making in trauma conversations. The categories of inquiry are shared here as they assist people to identify responses, foster the experience of personal agency, make visible skills and knowledge, and rehabilitate negative identity. This is what is possible in single session therapy, but this work takes a great deal of study and practice.[4] Also, there are many complimentary practices that can be part of these conversations that are beyond the scope of this chapter. Future focused or hypothetical future conversations[5] can provide a useful detour in meaning making. Externalizing practices and re-authoring certainly are useful depending on the scenario and fit. We bring all that we are and know to these conversations, holding the safety of the person at the centre of all we do.

Notes

1 By "trauma story" I am referring to when a story is shared involving a social or relational event(s) or trespass that is evocative, moving, and limiting the sharer's life. It is a subjective experience and can shape how people come to see themselves.

2 Michael White has referred to the therapist as the senior partner in the therapeutic encounter who facilitates the process assisting the participant to explore meaning favouring re-storying. Through a Vygotskian lens the therapist as the senior partner

provides questions that serve as a scaffolding assisting the participant to distance from the known and familiar first story moving towards what's possible to know and do. See White, M. 2007.

3 See Chapter 14 for a vignette example of a re-membering conversation in single session therapy.

4 I encourage you to read and study the work of those informing this chapter including White's work (2004), Angel Yuens' (2019), Wade (1997, 2002), and Vikki Reynolds (2020) to get started. While not specific to single session therapy their contributions are key and have influenced my conversations profoundly.

5 Hypothetical future conversations are thoroughly described in solution-focused brief therapy. See de Shazer et al., 2021; Dolan, 1991 for reference. There are many ways to enter into hypothetical future conversations and another great example is by David Epston (2008) as he describes a haunting from the future.

References

Batrouney, A. (2019). Narrative therapy approaches in single-session trauma work. *The International Journal of Narrative Therapy and Community Work*, (2), 40–48.

Beaudoin, M.-N. (2004). Problems with frogs, clients, and therapists: A cultural discourse analysis. *Journal of Systemic Therapies*, *23*(3), 51–63. https://doi.org/10.1521/jsyt.23.3.51.50755

Beaudoin, M.-N. (2005). Agency and choice in the face of trauma: A narrative therapy map. *Journal of Systemic Therapies*. *24*, 32–50. 10.1521/jsyt.2005.24.4.32.

Carey, M., Walther, S. & Russell, S. (2009). The absent but implicit: A map to support therapeutic enquiry. *Family Process*, *48*(3), 319–331. https://doi.org/10.1111/j.1545-5300.2009.01285.x

Clark, N. (2016). Shock and awe: Trauma as the new colonial frontier. *Humanities*, *5*(1), 1–16. https://doi.org/10.3390/h5010014

Denborough, D. (2008). *Strengthening resistance: The use of narrative practices in working with genocide survivors*. Adelaide, Australia: Dulwich Centre Publications.

de Shazer, S., Dolan, Y., Korman, H., Trepper, T., McCollum, E. & Berg, I. K. (2021). *More than miracles* (2nd ed.). Routledge.

Dolan, Y. (1991). *Resolving sexual abuse*. New York: Norton.

Epston, D., Cherelyn, L. & Tomm, K. (2008). Haunting from the future: A congenial approach to parent children conflicts. In B. Bowen (Ed.), *Down under and up over: Travels with narrative therapy* (pp. 97–109). AFT Pub.

Lumsden, R. (2020). Narrative approaches in a domestic violence hotline. *The International Journal of Narrative Therapy and Community Work*, (1), 2–9.

Malinen, T., Cooper, S. J. & Thomas, F. N. (Eds.). (2012). *Masters of narrative and collaborative therapies: The voices of Andersen, Anderson, & White*. New York: Routledge.

Marsten, D., Epston, D. & Markham, L. (2016). *Narrative therapy in wonderland: Connecting with children's imaginative know-how*. New York: W. W. Norton & Company.

Perdomo, C. (2017). Undocumented and deportable: Re-authoring trauma within the context of immigration in a narrative informed single session. *Journal of Systemic Therapies*, *36*(4), 3–15. https://doi.org/10.1521/jsyt.2017.36.4.3

Reynolds, V. (2020). Trauma and resistance: 'hang time' and other innovative responses to oppression, violence and suffering. *Journal of Family Therapy*. doi:10.1111/1467-6427.12293

Richardson, C. & Reynolds, V. (2014). Structuring safety in therapeutic work alongside indigenous survivors of residential schools. *The Canadian Journal of Native Studies, 34*(2), 147–164.

Strong, T. & Flynn, T. (2000). "Do you want this story to die with you?!" *Journal of Systemic Therapies, 19*(3), 83–88. https://doi.org/10.1521/jsyt.2000.19.3.83

Todd, N. & Wade, A. (2004). Coming to terms with violence and resistance: From a language of effects to a language of responses, in T. Strong & D. Pare (eds), *Furthering talk: Advances in the discursive therapies*. New York: Kluwer Academic Plenum.

Wade, A. (1997). Small acts of living: Everyday resistance to violence and other forms of oppression. *Contemporary Family Therapy, 19*(1), 23–39.

Wade, A. (2002). *From a language of effects to responses: Honouring our clients' resistance to violence*. New Therapist.

Wade, A. (2007). Despair, resistance, hope. In C. Flaskas, I. McCarthy & J. Sheehan (Eds.), *Hope and despair in narrative and family therapy: Adversity, forgiveness and reconciliation*. New York, NY: Routledge.

White, M. (2003). Narrative Practice and community assignments. *International Journal of Narrative Therapy and Community Work, 2003*(2): 17–55.

White, M. (2004). Working with people who are suffering the consequences of multiple trauma: A narrative perspective. *International Journal of Narrative Therapy and Community Work*, (1), 45–76. Reprinted in D. Denborough, (Ed.). (2006). *Trauma: Narrative responses to traumatic experience* (pp. 25–85). Adelaide, Australia: Dulwich Centre Publications.

White, M. (2005). Children, trauma and subordinate storyline development. *The International Journal of Narrative Therapy and Community Work, 2005*, 10.

White, M. & Morgan A. (2006). *Narrative therapy with children and their families*. Adelaide, South Australia: Dulwich Centre Publications.

Yuen, A. (2007). Discovering children's responses to trauma: a response-based narrative practice. *The International Journal of Narrative Therapy and Community Work, 2007*, 3.

Yuen, A. (2009). Less pain more gain: Explorations of responses versus effects when working with the consequences of trauma. *E-journal of narrative practice. 1*, 6–16. Dulwich Centre Foundation.

Yuen, A. (2019). *Pathways beyond despair: Re-authoring lives of young people through narrative therapy*. Adelaide, Australia: Dulwich Centre Publications.

Chapter 13

The Game Plan

To bring the brief narrative SST structure to life, I want to share a practice vignette. This story is an example of the kinds of trauma stories that are shared at the walk-in therapy clinic, as the participants' experience of pain and distress related to past events was so present in the room on this day.

Durene,[1] a 17-year-old female of Jamaican heritage, sat still and quiet in our waiting room. I arrived to greet her and welcome her to our meeting space. She hardly spoke but led the way to our meeting room as she had been to the clinic two weeks prior. Both these visits were encouraged by her child protection worker and the staff working at the transition home where she was living temporarily as they were concerned that she was "depressed".

Her pre-session paperwork shared very little as all questions were answered with "I don't know", including the question about what would be most important to talk about today. When I see these responses, I think about a few things. Could it be that the problem has made it difficult for the person to gain some distance from their life experience to enter into reflection? Could it be that there are dangers in talking about what they are experiencing? Could it be that they don't have the words to describe their experiences? Perhaps the pre-session questions are too big of a stretch from the familiar life they are living? Aside from these possibilities, her answers were a cue to me to remain curious, ask permission to ask my questions, and to seek a multi-storied conversation.

After brief introductions, I sought to learn from Durene why the service providers in her life wanted her to talk with me. She noted they thought she was sad, however her own view was that she just didn't like people or being around people. I asked how this view had come about, for instance, had she experienced people in ways that went against her beliefs about how to be in relationships? She confirmed this with the disclaimer that she had been through a lot in her life. Returning to the description of her as sad, I asked what made people think that was the case. She supposed it had to do with how much she preferred to be alone. In my mind, I was wondering if this described "sadness" and "wanting to be alone" could be a response to what she had been through in her life. I decided

DOI: 10.4324/9781003431688-14

not to ask about responses at this point in the conversation to hear more about her thoughts about her distress.

Trying to get oriented and to structure safety, I sought permission to ask further about what Durene linked to this sadness. She responded sharing her experience of a lifetime of being let down by people and specifically by her father. Durene then recounted a series of events through streaming tears. I was concerned by these tears, which seemed to flow without breaks between drops. She calmly wiped them aside with skill that suggested she had wiped tears aside countless times throughout her life. I gestured to the Kleenex, and she accepted this invitation to comfort after some time.

She carried on and shared a story of rejection and abuse from her father and a series of very difficult times that followed. She had found herself un-homed, cut off from family, and out of school. It was only when her fathers' ex-partner found out about her circumstances and contacted child protection services that Durene eventually found a home at a residence for youth who could no longer live with their families. She was continuing to get her education and doing well in this supportive setting.

First, I understand Durene's experience of distress related to her time with her father as a response that makes known the past circumstances are, in no way, okay with her. Second, sharing about those experiences represents an action. It's a step of separation from the distress it has caused her. I also understand that she must be discerning those experiences from implicit, not yet stated, preferences for a different life. Her sharing implied that, not only is she not okay with what has transpired in her life, but also that she holds a picture of the life she wants, including how relationships should be and perhaps more preferred ways of thinking about herself.

To learn more about these implicit storylines, I took a moment to enter into a brief response-based conversation. I shared back a short re-telling noting that it seemed to me she had been through a lot in the past few years. I invited her to consider if, in a sense, her experience of "wanting to be alone" was a response to what she had been though. She had supposed so. I asked what kind of response she had thought it was; did she consider it a way of protecting herself from future mistreatment and loss of relationships? Durene connected to this idea of protection noting she had resolved to never be in that situation again. I wondered if this was like taking a cautious approach to life and people. Durene hadn't thought of it as an approach before, but this made sense to her.

A second story had begun to come visible in which Durene was not depressed and isolating as a symptom of Depression but rather taking a cautious approach to life and relationships to ensure a safer path. She added that she actually has one friend with whom she is hoping to move in with so she can be closer to her community and culture. To me, as the theme of "a cautious approach" emerged, Durene was now starting to recall events more fitting the emerging second story.

I wondered what her experience of sadness might speak to about what was important to her that she was seeking out in life. She supposed this too connected to her longing for safety and kindness in life. Was it like a way of saying this has to change, I'm not where I want to be in life and relationships? Again, she had supposed so and we talked about sadness as a longing for things to be different. Understanding her distress as an act of separation and to canvas her preferred future that she was longing for, I decided to invite Durene to explore a future focused story. These stories move forward through the timeline, speculating about events on a landscape of action while weaving through speculation on the landscape of identity and place. They canvas the imagination and draw out prospective knowledge.

I invited Durene to picture in her minds' eye time travelling five years into the future towards her preferred life. Once she arrived at the imaginary time period, I asked questions that had her acquaint me with her preferred future. She told how she will be working, providing for herself, be able to take care of herself and helping her mother out. She would have her own place to live and might be open more to people, evidenced by connecting with a friend for lunch. She would have finished her education and have a sense of happiness and "smooth sailing in life".

Turning to the landscape of meaning within this future-focused story, I asked what she would be knowing more fully about herself in that future? Durene, now seeming to be able to adopt a more reflexive stance, oscillating throughout the timeline, highlighted that she "is strong, can endure a lot of things and know who she is in the end". At this point, I chose not to learn more about the historical and relational aspects of her "strength" to learn more about other things her future self will have learned.

She continued in the present sighting, "I have a lot of abilities; how to ground myself and stay focused on the path to what I am reaching for". This last sentiment caught my attention as a metaphor of movement, and I wanted to explore it further through co-creating a take-away document. I asked Durene if it would be okay if I showed her on a piece of paper what was coming to mind for me. With her approval, I drew the three domains of the "rites of passage" metaphor and shared the following summary.

Durene, I have this image of you reaching for the life you want, taking a cautious approach and this has me thinking about the path you have been on. Here on this paper is how we draw these paths in life. This first section represents what you are moving away from, what was no longer okay with you, what you are separating from. Given that you are moving away from this, you must be moving towards your vision of what you are reaching for, as you have said. This third area represents where you are headed. So, the middle part is the journey or path with its storms and detours, etc. If you think of this as your path, where would you put yourself currently? For instance, are you still at the beginning in those tough times with your dad or are you on the path?

Durene indicated she was at the beginning of the middle part. I continued, "Okay, so you are not back at the beginning, but have already started on the path, if I am getting this right?" Durene confirmed this was correct. Extending the journey metaphor further and building on her "smooth sailing" metaphor, I wondered if her current residence was like a safe harbour from the storms and a place to get ready for the journey ahead. She confirmed that it was as the metaphor continued to fit for her. To archive what we were learning and to continue to bring the metaphor into focus I asked if we could take some time to fill in the document with some details.

Durene accepts this invitation and in the "separation" domain draws her dad as well as writes the words "My Mind". She explains to me how these words represent how the past can get her thinking "there is no hope" or that she "is not loved or cared about" and that these ideas can try to hold her back. She links this to the lens her father had, as he would often say negative things about her and to her. I invited her to name this first domain, and she assigned the title "The Challenger".

As is often the process, once people identify what they are separating from, there is a natural jump to discussing where they wish to arrive; the third phase of the rites of passage. Durene named the future third phase "Smooth Sailing in the Future" and included images representing her own house, her education, interests in fashion and design, peaceful times, as well as a reconnection with her Jamaican culture. She noted where she was currently living is primarily in a white community and she is looking to get back to the urban centre where she can reconnect to her culture as it "helps to feel connected to who you are".

Lastly, I invited Durene to explore the space on the document between where she was and where she was headed. She named this space "The Game Plan". I inquired as to what skills, abilities, and know-how she imagined would be good to keep with her on this journey or to pack in her suitcase, so to speak. Durene highlighted several ideas, including concepts such as hope, education, determination, strength, and the ability to self-advocate. She also identified current relationships. Those included a staff at her current home and a friend who would be useful to keep along the way to shoulder her up when things got difficult or if she started to lose her way.

We had arrived at a point in which we had travelled a fair distance in this conversation. At this point, Durene appeared much more animated, and the tears had subsided a while ago. Her document was complete for today, however, I sought to learn how she would consult this document and the difference it might make to her when she left. Her plan was to keep this Game Plan on her wall in her

Rites of Passage Map

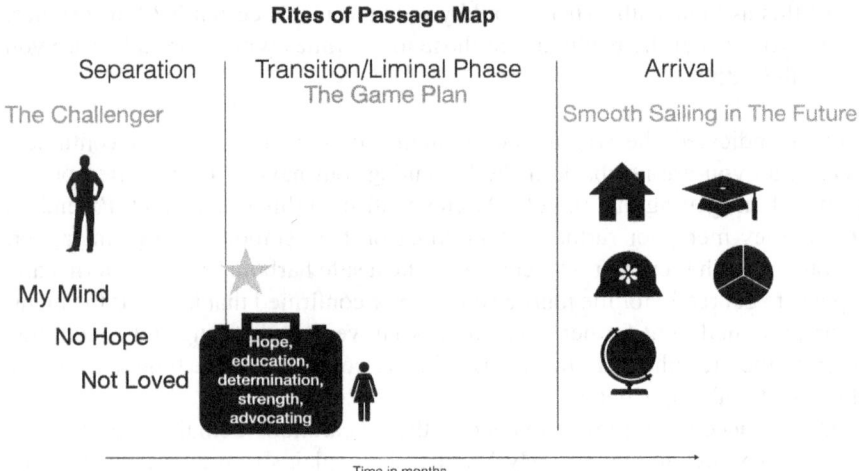

Figure 13.1 This is the pictorial representation of Durenes' journey. Co-creating a visual representation is often useful for people to situate and remember the important parts of the conversation.

residence and to look at it daily for some time. She noted it helped to continue to "understand where [she] is going because no matter what happens, seeing the end goal makes the obstacles not worth focusing on". Shortly after this conversation Durene moved out of the residence and in with the friend closer to her culture and preferred community.

Whereas Durene had been encouraged to come to the walk-in to address what people in her life were calling "her depression", the story-in-the-making that emerged was very different. Understanding her experience of distress as an act of separation and sadness as a longing for things to be different, assisted Durene to come to know herself as active in her life. She had a vision of the life she was seeking, was taking a cautious approach, and mapping this journey assisted it to come more in focus.

Note

1   Durene is a pseudonym and details have been altered to respect confidentiality.

Chapter 14

Re-membering Conversations

Facing Cancer

Single session conversations can be very moving. I have had the fortune to meet several children and youth who were experiencing extreme grief regarding the loss of a loved one to cancer. I meet these children and youth when what they are experiencing has become unbearable and limits their daily living. They may no longer enjoy restful sleep. They may no longer wish to engage with the world, avoiding school, friends, and family. Conversation reveals a profound sense of loss.

Conversation also reveals the significantly revised roles children and youth step into, responding to their loved one as they tried to survive the illness. Many aspects of these roles involved foregoing what they would usually have been doing, such as attending school, sports, or playing with friends, to adopt roles in closer proximity to their suffering loved one. I've heard accounts of regular hospital visits, switching in with adults to care take, sit with, or the deliver various treatments. I've heard how many youth take to monitoring or providing ways to comfort or distract their loved one from pain in the face of suffering from the side effects of treatments. I've also heard stories of how children carried on as usual despite their preference to remain at home and with their loved one, respecting their loved ones' wishes. The broader illness narrative of suffering and sense of loss often eclipses this range of responses. They only come visible when sought through respectful inquiry and further developed with the re-membering conversation map (White, 1997, 2007, 2011).

Re-membering conversations in these situations first trace what the loved one contributed to the youths' life. I inquire how the youth came to know themselves through their relationship; often as loved, cared about, important, the sun and the moon, meaning everything, etc. Second, and typically a more novel conversation for the child/youth is inquiring about what they may have contributed to the loved one's life and how might that loved one have come to know themselves through the relationship with the child/youth. Often responses include as a good parent, loved, knowing their teachings will live on through the child, etc.

DOI: 10.4324/9781003431688-15

Regarding loss from illness such as cancer, it has seemed useful to focus the conversation, in part, around the youth's contribution while the loved one navigated medical treatment through to their death. That timeline often reveals astonishing skills and very meaningful contributions to the loved one's life.

Regarding the loved one witnessing a youth carry on as usual during their illness, we may come to learn how that was reassuring to the dying person. Witnessing the child/youth, they may have come to be reassured that the child would be fine after they have passed. It perhaps lets them know they had done a wonderful job as a parent. Knowing that might have been extremely comforting in their final days and hours of life. Upon considering this, the youth may experience a revised understanding of their parent's last hours and an appreciation of the legacy of skills and hopes for their future left to them. That may invite a re-engagement with life that honours their loved one through each future action.

When skills of "care taking" and "comforting" are foregrounded, I learn about how the figure may have come to know how deeply they were loved. They may have experienced pride in witnessing their offspring's skills, courage, and love. It can be speculated that witnessing this may have assisted a parent to know again that they had done well. Often, it can be speculated that this comfort may have helped the parent to hold out, fight the disease longer, and soak up every last minute of living a life.

To honour and become more richly acquainted with this account, again, is honouring of the loved one and often experienced as comforting to the youth. To know and understand their contribution in this way provides a revised storyline related to the death.

References

White, M. (1997). Re-membering. In M. White *Narratives of therapists' lives,* Adelaide: Dulwich Centre Publications.

White, M. (2007). *Maps of narrative practice.* New York: W.W. Norton.

White, M. (2011). *Narrative practice: Continuing the conversations.* New York: W.W. Norton.

Chapter 15

Single Session Therapy and Crisis Conversations

Many people attend the walk-in clinic who consider themselves as "in crisis", indicating they are at risk of death by suicide, engaging in self-injury, or experiencing emotions as overwhelming. While single session conversations at the walk-in or by appointment are not meant as replacements for crisis services that provide personal risk assessment, there is a great deal we can accomplish while simultaneously shoring up safety. This chapter outlines options for navigating risk conversations in single session therapy. Extending the analogy of the rites of passage, we understand the experience of crisis as an important transition. As such, we can talk about the experience of crisis differently, fostering revised understandings and hope for the future. Eminent danger should always take precedent and be responded to prudently.

Many therapists experience tension when they meet with people at the walk-in who express a compromised sense of personal safety, overwhelming life circumstances, and/or struggle to see the possibilities for their future. I have heard colleagues question why the walk-in was recommended to people as opposed to crisis services. It can reflect a struggle to know how to navigate these conversations. It can also reflect the thought that the person needs more than a single session.

I recognize these conversations can be messy, that is, slow to progress and where it's difficult to know how to proceed. You may hear one-word answers and be meeting with people with little affect. Other times, it may be difficult to nudge the conversation out of the mire of the problem story. Despite this, these conversations have the potential for life-changing ripples. Moments of perceived crisis are a reflection of change-in-motion and rich in possibility. When we meet people in these moments and work to learn about alternate story, new possibilities emerge.

Risk Assessment

As it's an ongoing process throughout the therapeutic conversation, we do not administer risk assessment through a standardized device or tool. We do not stop

DOI: 10.4324/9781003431688-16

the therapeutic conversation to administer such a tool. While these tools direct attention towards perceived level of risk intended to alert the therapist to take up the project of safety planning, they simultaneously direct attention away from safety. Risk assessment is not seen as a separate event within our time together. It is an ongoing process of meaning making through dialogue, learning about and discussing risks, while also tending to safety through the threading of the story-in-the-making.

Risk assessment begins within the pre-session paperwork as we ask participants to indicate if they are at risk of harm to themselves or someone else. Should they check off that box, it alerts the therapist to ask further questions. However, should they not check off that box, there are storylines we are listening for that alert the therapist to ask questions discerning risk and safety.

Defining Risk

From an outside vantage point "In crisis" is difficult to define, yet clear-cut definitions are often pursued to match a service to the situation. When we are working with perception and meaning, definitions are more ambiguous than precise. However, to make risk visible, I am guided by the following modified from Lipchik (2002):

- Expressions of a danger of physical harm to self or others.
  Ex) I'm suicidal, I don't want to be here anymore, I wish I were dead.
- Expressions perceived by someone other than the person (including therapist) of danger to self or someone else.
  Ex) I could cut until I can't cut anymore, I just have to be back together with my girlfriend.
- Expressions of self-perceived lack of control over emotions.
  Ex) I just can't stop crying, I wish I would never wake up again.

With this loose definition, I have found it useful to have some markers to flag for the therapist storylines of risk and storylines that may have people vulnerable to compromised safety. In understanding risk shaped by a post-structural sentiment, SST conversations in which the person experiences any of the following alerts me to address safety.

Limiting Stories

Stories we hold about ourselves can limit what experiences get noticed and taken into storylines. Some grand narratives have people more vulnerable to death by suicide. Familiarizing with these plot lines helps us hear them as a warning that safety may be vulnerable, compromised, or fleeting. Some of these plot lines can include:

- A storied sense of personal burden to those they care about.
- An eclipsed vision of the possibilities that lie ahead for one's life.
- Conclusions about who one is such as worthless, a failure, unlovable.
- A theme of compromised belonging and connection.
- A theme of no way out of a situation, such as a sense of being trapped or oppressed.
- A plot of hopelessness, little sense of an ability to influence the situation paired with no ideas about what to do.

Contextual Concerns

Context can also play a part in rendering people vulnerable to harm and risk. Reynolds, V. (2012) exposes this locating suicide through a social justice perspective resisting "the individualism of suicide" (p. 2). In our single session conversations, I am on the lookout for contexts that disadvantage people or are frankly harmful and oppressive. When these situations become visible, the therapist may be required to take action outside the single session. With participants' permission we can provide advocacy and play a part in addressing the circumstance. Some contexts of concern may include:

- Relational isolation; cut off from culture, community, spirituality, and relationships through spatial and social separation.
- The means/ability to carry out an act such as access to weapons, pills, knives, etc.
- Severe oppression through relationship, social structures, institutional structures, political violence, poverty, racism, heterosexual dominance, exploitation, etc.
- Past attempts and loss of family members by suicide.
- An impoverished circle of care/support.

In SST, our time with someone may be the first and last time we meet with them. Given this, there are some important considerations relevant to doing our best to shore up safety and provide a conversation that is useful to people.

A. Working with Meaning Making:

Lipchik (2002) notes the "… therapist must recognize that he or she is a participant in the co-construction of the meaning of the crisis and also its possible resolution" (p. 199). As noted, working within the realm of meaning generation is a central project in brief narrative therapy. As such, new meanings can be co-developed and old meanings re-negotiated that are more supportive and sustaining of safety. My aim is to get on to story lines that are hope friendly, protective, and sustaining. These storylines involve the notion of "movement in life" opposing stuck-ness, personal agency opposing helplessness and possibility opposing futility.

B. Escape the Tyranny of the Binary:

In conceiving of the expression of "in crisis" as a moment or stop off on the journey of life, binary thinking no longer applies. Escaping binary views of "in crisis" versus "not in crisis" allows for multiple meanings, experiences, and identities to be considered and discussed (Fook, 2002, p. 13). Escaping a binary understanding of in crisis orients us to explore with people the liminal space as part of the rites of passage analogy. It is that space between thresholds of separation and arrival. This phase is described as the "betwixed and between" status and role (Turner & Bruner, 1986). It helps us to understand that someone arriving noting they are "suicidal" does not reflect a fixed static state.

C. Contextualize Distress:

Many will come to see their distress as an aberration of their brain reflecting a personal deficit or flaw in who they are. That can be a very limiting understanding as it backgrounds not only what people have been through, but also the many ways they have been responding to their circumstances. It leaves out the ways they have held on or carried on despite the context of their lives, which may have included disadvantage, poverty, judgment, racism, or mistreatment. When we learn about the context of people's distress, their experiences begin to make more sense to them and are located out in the world. Their conclusions reached, given these experiences, can then be discussed and linked. New ways of proceeding may then come available.

D. Safety Plan at or Near the End of the Session:

Although safety issues are foremost, the time to safety plan is negotiable and many times in SST it's most useful to safety plan near or at the end of the broader therapeutic conversation. The reason being is it's anticipated that by the end of the session, the person may know themselves and the situation differently. In that revised space, new options for proceeding come available to consider and employ. For example, as a problem is externalized and related to context rather than assumed to be a fault in one's mind, previously discounted options for proceeding come visible. Thus, the co-developed safety plan may look significantly different than if it had been developed at the beginning of the session.

E. Co-develop Safety Plans:

As we do our safety planning nearing the end of the session, we can invite participants into co-creating safety plans that are contextually relevant and in harmony with the developing storylines and identity status. This is a means to shore up safety through the liminal phase of the rite of passage; a phase often experienced as confusing, difficult, and complex as one moves towards and through unfamiliar status and ideas about how to be in the world. Safety plans are informed by the participant, archived for them in their own words, and given to them in a take-away document. These safety plans highlight what the person can do to keep themselves safe and external controls or others that can play a part in that safety.

There is space on the Conversation Summary to note the safety plan. I usually jump off the Conversation Summary and co-develop a separate safety plan document. The benefit of this is we are creating a document that can be copied and shared and posted where it would be most useful, untethered from the broader summary. I invite a title specific to this plan as well. If you were to give this plan a title, what would it be? People share titles they will remember and reflect an experience near definition such as, My Plan to Protect My Future, Keeping Safety Safe, My Road Map to the Life I Want.

F. Personal Agency and/or External Control:

We are always looking to facilitate conversations in which people experience personal agency. I strive to ask questions that assist people to experience a sense that they have say over their life, and that they can affect their life and circumstances. We have explored many kinds of questions that foster agency throughout this book, such as those within the landscape of action seeking exceptions and initiatives, "how" questions, and questions eliciting peoples' know-how. This is not to say that at times external supports who provide external safety are not needed. External supports can be an important part of the circle of care.

G. Shore up Circles of Care:

With the person(s) involved, we co-identify and co-create circles of care, including people who will shoulder up the person in distress and assist with ensuring safety should the distress become overwhelming or the journey too treacherous. These people can include close relations, friends, and professionals who may play a temporary part in helping. We can explore what role people can provide and link to local crisis services that can provide 24-hour availability for consultation or more formal risk assessment. It may mean activating local authorities to assist people for whom risk is too dominating.

Who is your best friend, someone who has stuck by you through thick and thin? What is your guess about what it is they see in you that has them hanging in there? What might they come to say they appreciate most about you? Would they be someone who stands for your future and the possibilities for your life? What part could they play in shouldering you up when things get tough? How often should they connect with you throughout the day?

H. Re-conceptualizing Crisis as a Transition:

For single session conversations, I have found a re-conceptualization of "in crisis" most useful in providing entry points to difference and possibility. White and Epston (1990) propose understanding the experience of crisis as relating to "...some aspect of a transition in a person's life" (p. 7). This transition can be both a shift in someone's role and a shift in how someone knows themselves and relates to their world. This is a move away from a more traditional understanding shaped by positivist sciences that identify the experience of crisis as a breakdown or malfunction of a person's coping. Understanding the experience of crisis as a transition in life, we are oriented once again by the analogy of the "rite of passage" and the three phases of separation, liminal, and reincorporation (Van Gennep, 1960; Turner, 1969).

The rite of passage analogy shapes several kinds of questions available to us in a single session for risk assessment and safety planning. White and Epston (1990, p.8) highlight several domains of inquiry informed by these phases that

... invite persons to determine (a) what the crisis might be telling them about what they could be separating from that was not viable for them—perhaps certain negative attitudes that they have towards themselves or that others have towards them, or expectations and prescriptions for their life and relationships that they experience as impoverishing; (b) what clues the crisis gives about the new status and roles that could become available to them (c) when, how, and under what circumstances these new roles and status might be realized.

Let's look more closely at each phase as it relates to these ideas. I have included a vignette of a young adult to share what kind of conversations are possible.

a. Separation

Having to do with shifts in identity and/or role, the separation phase suggests a departure from the way things are. It's a movement in life towards a revised identity and/or preferred role in life and relationships. The experience and expression of distress marks the separation phase. Often, what gets understood as symptoms can be understood as the act of separation. As such, it's a movement, response, and action representing separation. "People are not just giving a passive re-telling of what is problematic, rather the expression of the problem can itself be thought of as a response" (Carey, Walther & Russell, 2009, p.7).

This action is founded on people's intentions for their life. In hearing expressions of distress as actions, we are once again invoking Whites' concept of the absent but implicit (White, 2003). We can be curious about what this action implies that they are moving towards and away from–the intention of it.

Kendra, a 16-year-old identifying as they/them youth, attended the walk-in clinic accompanied by their father and stepmother. They struck me as mature for their age, insightful and composed. The adults had noted they had suffered "a breakdown" and may need some psychiatric treatment and medication, but they had thought they would have them seen at the walk-in as a first step. Kendra had indicated on the pre-session paperwork that they were at risk of harm to themself.

Both caregivers sited Kendra had a long history of "anxiety" and "depression" throughout their childhood. The "break down" was a sign for them, confirming Kendra needed to begin ongoing therapy. They had learned about the walk-in through their recent admission to the local hospital emergency room. Understandably, the focus of the youth and caregivers was on the significance of the breakdown, which was described as uncontrollable emotion, crying, and anger following a breakup with a boyfriend and the subsequent experience of emotional abuse and threat to expose private texts to their peers.

The most recent "break down" came following a phone call from their ex-partner who engaged in verbal threat and guilting. They had experienced this far too often in the relationship. Following this phone experience, they felt overwhelmed, helpless, and at fault for the relationship ending.

By the time Kendra arrived at the walk-in clinic, they had had several conversations regarding the breakdown and the extent to which they were "at risk" to themself. Safety plans had been developed and shared with Kendra, including monitoring by their caregivers. The extent of these conversations remained limited in that they were in relation to the incident and what it meant about their "mental status". Those domains of inquiry, while important, can contribute to shaping a spoiled identity (Goffman, 1963). That is, a sense of the problem as a reflection of broken or malfunctioning parts of the person, an aberration of their brain or illness.

Kendra's distress, named a "breakdown", inferring something has broken in them, evidences this understanding and consequently limits the responses to the world available to them. In this scenario, options were limited to the idea that medication can correct the breakage or psychiatric treatment will fix what's wrong.

What had been understood as a "breakdown" when viewed through the rite of passage analogy represents the beginning of a transformation, moving away from "what has been", as those circumstances were no longer viable for Kendra. The breakdown can be understood as an action in the form of a response, protesting mistreatment and a future of more of the same. Kendra was striving to separate from a harmful relationship and unwelcome ways of seeing themself. The journey ahead wasn't clear and was somewhat into the unknown.

Understanding this, I offered many questions for Kendra to consider. What does their distress speak to about what has happened that is not okay with them or bumps up against their values? How does what they experienced go against their ideas about how people should treat each other? What might their distress indicate about what they stand against and what they stand for? What has this experience tried to have them think about themself that doesn't fit well for them? If their distress was thought of as a response of some kind, what kind of response might it be; a protest, a way of saying I'm not okay with this situation, a way to not let this person off the hook for their mistreatment?

These questions seemed to reorient Kendra to their values and beliefs about how relationships should be. As they considered their distress as an action, they noted that, "It's saying his actions are abusive and not okay and I will not suffer in silence with it." They highlighted how important trust is to them in a relationship and how it had been so deeply breeched.

As is often the case, discussion about what someone is separating from jumps to discussion of the preferred destination. I then come back to discuss the liminal space that they have entered.

b. Liminal

Struggle, confusion, disorganization, and discomfort often accompanies the liminal phase. This is a place in which we see people struggle, sometimes for a long time. It is a time in which they are seeking clarity, becoming, and exploring what might be. It can be particularly disruptive as one's place and/or identity comes under review and revision. A person may be wrestling with the gap between how they view themselves and their preferred view. The greater the gap, the greater the distress.

The liminal phase, as territory to travel across, involves the steps people are required to take to arrive somewhere more preferred. We can be curious about what these steps might be and the pros and cons of them. We can be curious about markers along the way and signs of progress.

As Kendra's story demonstrates, they had a clear wish to separate from what they had been through and was, to some degree, still experiencing. They had entered a space in which they were struggling to know which way was up in relationships, so to speak. This was an unsettling space, with some serious fears for what might come next should he release the private texts or continue to call. I asked questions with the hope they could assist them to navigate this space, experience agency, and recognize progress along the way.

Kendra, if we think about this as a storm of sorts that has come through your life (they corrected the metaphor to a hurricane) what are your ideas about how to protect yourself in this situation? What's important to remember about yourself in this situation? What difference will it make to keep that in your heart as you weather this?

Despite their distress, Kendra came up with some practical steps they could take to protect themselves, including blocking on social media, limiting social media, and doing the things that bring them joy. They highlighted the importance of remembering they are loved and have many people in their life who would stand with them against such a trespass. They shared stories about other past contributions to their life. This thinking was likened to shielding from the hail and winds trying to unearth them.

c. Reincorporation

The reincorporation phase within a crisis conversation is somewhat in the realm of imagination, speculation, and hypothetical future. It represents a preferred life and preferred view of self. It is the place where people wish to arrive. To know separation, one must have a sense of what they want different. To have a sense of what they want different, they must have experienced it previously, seen an example at some point, or imagined a preferred future. We can bring this material into the conversation in meaningful ways. Importantly, by asking about a more preferred future implies this future is possible. These questions, while speculative and hypothetical, are, for the most part, phrased as pre-suppositional, implying this will come to be.

As noted, Kendra had a clear understanding of what they were separating from which implies they have a view of a more preferred destination. We explored this vision together. I wondered what their ideas were about the kind of relationship they were seeking? At what times had they experienced a relationship more in harmony with that vision? When they have come through this hurricane and had "rebuilt" (their emerging metaphor), what will they be knowing about themself that this experience had tried to have them question? How will they be treating themself and thinking about themself in this future? What lessons would they have learned that they would turn into advice for their future daughter or friends? Was this a wisdom they were growing?

At this point in the conversation, new storylines are emerging. One reflects a revised identity, the movement from being broken or breaking down to responding, weathering a hurricane, and taking actions founded on important values. The context related to their experience of distress is more visible. Rather than an internal failure on their part now requiring psychiatric repair, the focus is on addressing abuse and creating a safer world.

Following this conversation, nearing the end of the session, and from this revised sense of identity, I invited Kendra to reflect on checking the box "at risk to self" in the pre-session paperwork. I asked, "If 10 out of 10 is I'm completely safe and 1 is the opposite of that, where would you place yourself right now?"

They replied, "Well, after we have been talking about this, I would say I'm at a 9/10." They noted the worst it had been was a 1/10 a few days prior when "things were really bad and it was everyday".

This presented a good time to co-craft a safety plan to maintain their current sense of safety. This was a means to assist them to continue to weather the hurricane as they would be returning home to a context in which they still may experience judgement from peers or unwelcome texts.

Safety Planning

This process does not preclude the co-development of safety plans. My understanding is that Problems can make comebacks and the various receiving contexts of people's lives for meaning can be highly constraining, making it difficult to proceed in some circumstances. For example, when Kendra returns home, it is likely the ex-partner will try to contact them. Given this, it is important to co-craft safety plans that are meaningful and context specific.

There are some important aspects to safety plans. As noted, in SST we tend to safety plan near the end of the session. When the time is right, safety plans are co-developed, meaning we share in the creation of them eliciting participants' ideas and suggestions alongside proposing our own resources and ideas in a tentative voice. Plans ideally foreground the participant taking action to grow their safety as opposed to reliance solely on external controls ensuring safety.

This does not mean external controls such as supportive allies may not be called upon or the participant be routed to the emergency room. These external temporary controls may be important and warranted however we balance them with actions the participant will take to grow safety. Safety plans also engage allies who can be there to help shoulder the person up as needed and play a part in ensuring safety. Ideally, this is done by inviting the participant to identify these people and plan together how they could be involved. Often, people are connected to crisis services who can provide ongoing support as needed.

Our crisis services run parallel to all our services and people can move in and out of them as needed. Often, we will facilitate introducing participants to a crisis service provider when possible. Other times, we will gain permission for the crisis service to reach out to the participant later that day as a step in the plan. Lastly, these plans are documented as a take-away document. As with any take-away document, I ask participants to give the document a name and we discuss where to keep it and when to consult it.

Returning to our point of reference questions, I asked Kendra, "At what number would it be important to tell someone close to you so that they could play their part in shouldering you up should you need that?"

They shared that should their sense of safety drop to a 5 it would be important for them to share it with their mother and they were agreeable to do so.

"Okay, so on your safety plan should I write that down; something like, if safety drops to a five, I will let my mom know?"

"Yes, sure that sounds good."

I asked who else was part of their life club[1]; those who stand with them in their values and stand for their future. They identified four others who could be included in their circle of care that could be called upon if needed. We explored potential times to call on them and the various specific parts they could play. Kendra was provided with the crisis service information should they also like to talk to someone when others aren't available. This plan was documented, and then Kendra consulted to me about who to share the plan with and where they would keep it, so it was there when they needed it. They named the plan "Weather Proofing My Life".

Conceiving of the expression of distress as an action within the broader journey of separation, transition, and arrival assists people to move away from the idea of distress as a personal flaw. Questions oriented by the rite of passage helped to navigate this conversation simultaneously assessing risk while languaging into existence possibility and safety. The following are possible questions related to this idea that the expression of distress/crisis is an action suggesting a preferred destination and are organized according to the phases of the rites of passage.

Separation Phase

Questions about separation:

- What might this distress/crisis be telling you that you are separating from; that you want to be different? (Something no longer viable or negative attitudes they have towards themselves.)
- Are there certain expectations or prescriptions for your life that no longer sit well with you?
- What is the first sign this journey has begun?
- What is it you need to keep with you or around you as you take these steps to bring your future more in harmony with your wishes?
- How are you going to take care as you figure this out? Who else could play a part in this care or shoulder you up as you go?

Questions about separating from identity conclusions:

- What no longer works for you in seeing yourself that way; as depressed?
- When do you know yourself in other, more preferred ways?
- How would you like to be thinking about yourself and your life?
- How would you like people to know you?
- When are you seeing that these ideas about life and who you are do not speak the whole truth about you and who you are becoming?
- As you begin to revise this understanding about yourself, what will you come to know more of/ less of?

Questions about separating from role and/or context:

- What about this relationship no longer fits with your hopes or dreams?
- What are your ideas about the kind of relationships you are now seeking out and what are you deciding to leave behind?
- Who have you known previously in which you have experienced what you are seeking? Who taught you about that?
- What is it about this situation that no longer fits with what you want in your life?
- What about this situation are you now looking at leaving or separating from? What are you seeking out?

Liminal Phase

Questions about learning along the way:

- What might be the first sign that your journey has begun; that things are improving?
- What might you be starting to do/think differently?
- What might you be starting to know differently about yourself/your life?
- Who might be around? Where might you be living?
- What will be a sign to you that things are on track, more how you want them to be?
- Tell me about a time when you've taken a step like this before? How did you make that happen?
- What's in it for you along the way?
- What might be something that tries to have you veer off course?
- Should the way become foggy or hard to see, who would you call upon for guidance?
- What are your fears should this transition begin to unfold? How will you muster your bravery should the fears try to hold you back?

Reincorporation Phase

Questions about a preferred future:

- What is it that you want to be different?
- What's this distress say about the kind of life you want?
- Tell me about what you'd like different in your life or relationships?
- How will you be thinking about yourself differently than you are now?
- How will you celebrate your success? Who will it be important to include in that celebration?
- What circumstances will be in place that let you know you have arrived?
- Imagine we meet again in a year and this distress/situation has passed. What might you be thinking differently about yourself, doing differently? What might be happening in your life that is currently absent?

Supporting Practices

The brief therapies offer many useful kinds of questions to assist people experiencing crisis to foreground experiences that we can bring into stories-in-the-making. Here are a few, in no particular order. This list is also not exhaustive but highlights a few domains of inquiry that nudge the conversation towards protective storylines and foreground reasons for living and possibility.

Point of Reference Questions (Qualitative and Quantitative Scaling)

Any journey can be assisted by having points of reference from which to discern direction and place. Point of reference questions in the form of subjective scaling (popularized by de Shazer et al.) can assist to orient to the here and now and mark points of progress along the journey. Difference can quickly be ascertained in contrasting these points of reference.

For example, 10/10 is I will leave here and follow through with killing myself and 1/10 is the opposite, where would you scale yourself in this moment, when you arrived, the worst it's been, the best? At what number would it be important to tell someone that you are experiencing compromised safety? Should we meet again in a few days, and you tell me you have moved up the scale even a little bit? What will you be thinking differently?

Externalizing Practices

Externalizing concepts such as hopelessness, discouragement, and failure assists people to make visible the ways Problems try to influence their life and thinking. In the vignette, Kendra discussed "The Hurricane" that had come into their life. Discussion about the ways these problems develop and go about their business begins to render the person as the protagonist in their own life and the Problem as the antagonist. As such, the protagonist can begin to adjust their relationship with the problem and reflect on times when the antagonist was less dominating. This juxtaposition can muster an impassioned position to carry on and the conversation provides opportunity for the protagonists' own initiatives and know-how to become more visible. Further, as previously noted in Chapter 11, externalizing conversations bring context into the conversation, making visible oppression, injustice, and mistreatment to be addressed, as opposed to locating the problem in the person as some malfunction to be fixed.

> How is it you have been able to carry on despite what Hopelessness has tried to get you to focus on? What kind of things does Hopelessness try to get you to think and believe? How is it you have hung on to the future possibilities for your life despite Hopelessness' tactics? What is happening that has invited Hopelessness into your life?

Response-based Conversations

An expression of distress understood as an action can be viewed more specifically as a response (Wade, 1997, 2002; Todd & Wade, 2004; Reynolds, 2020). These are conversations that recognize and foreground people's responses to experiences of hardship, trespass, or oppression. Expressions are viewed as "resistance" (Reynolds, 2020) to the way things are or ways of saying they are no longer complicit with circumstances. Often, those responses are understood as symptoms of some underlying illness or deficit. Recognizing responses rather than symptoms not only provides clues to the early stages of the rite of passage but provides ways of talking about distress that put it in a new light.

> What if we think of this distress as a response to what you have been experiencing? What kind of response would you say it is; a protest, a refusal to be complicit with or silent about what you have been through? What values or beliefs does that say are important to you about relationships/the world, etc.?

Focus on Difference

Crisis storylines leave a great deal of lived life out of the picture. We can ask about initiatives and exceptions, invite attribution of significance, and bring into stories-in-the-making that sustain people long after the session. Getting on to meaningful difference in these conversations can be the "difference that makes a difference" (Bateson, 1972, p. 453). These questions, too, benefit from a pre-suppositional phrasing that assumes difference.

> When the thoughts of suicide come, how long do they stay? What are you doing to make them go away (Fiske, H., 2008)? Tell me about a time when you were thinking differently? What were you thinking/doing at that time? Tell me about a time when things weren't as bad? How did you make that happen? I imagine there were times when this problem could have got the best of you in the past, however you defied it. How did you do that? What is a small sign that things are more on track? How did you manage to go that long between attempts? How did you stop yourself from cutting deeper?

Coping (Problem Refusal)

People are always taking actions to carry on despite what they are up against. We can conceive of these actions as refusals to let the Problem dominate them. Inquiring about these acts, whether they be counter thoughts, feelings, or actions, can provide the material to build upon into ongoing safety plans and reacquaint people with their ability to direct their life in the face of any circumstance.

> Given all that you have been through, how is it you have been able to carry on this long? What does that say about you and what you want different for your future? How come you are not resigned to this life? What keeps you going even in the most difficult times? How come things aren't worse?

Future Focused Stories

This includes questions to evoke the imagination and move away from entrenched thinking, oppressive storylines, or hopelessness. This can include hypothetical future questions (de Shazer et al., 1986; Epston, Lakusta & Tomm, 2008). These questions typically invite people into exploration of a hypothetical future not yet realized yet possible and not linearly related to the "crisis" material.

> Suppose we were to meet five years from now and things were better, what would you say made the difference? Suppose when you walk through this door to go home all the problems that led to you meeting with me are gone. What would be different? Suppose we were visited right now from a future you who had gotten through this time, what would they say to bring you relief and hope?

A storied hypothetical future explores and links the material informed by the dual landscapes in a re-authoring conversation. Landscape of action refers to the hypothetical preferred events and landscape of identity to the sense people make of these events as they relate to who they hypothetically are becoming.

> Suppose that was to happen. How might you come to know yourself differently? When you take that step, what might it suggest even a little bit to you about what might be possible for your life?

A storied account of a hypothetical future is compelling, languaging into existence a possible future.

Reasons for Living

Assisting people to articulate reasons for living (Fiske, 2008) provides material for compelling counter-stories to distress and worthlessness. Eliciting details of answers to these questions serves to assist the emerging counter story to become durable.

> What keeps you going? …helps you push back those darkness? If there was one thing that might be worth living for right now, what would it be? What kept you alive when you felt this way before?

This chapter extends the analogy of the rites of passage to conceptualizing the experience of crisis. This proves useful in introducing new avenues for inquiry in the context of single session brief narrative therapy. This is a move away from the sole employment of external controls to achieve safety towards processes that support the development and experience of personal agency. We assess risk all along the way in these therapeutic conversations as we explore risk and safety together.

Note

1 See Chapter 17 for an explanation of the "life club" metaphor.

References

Bateson, G. (1972). *Steps to an ecology of mind*. New York: Chandler.

Carey, M., Walther, S. & Russell, S. (2009). The absent but implicit: A map to support therapeutic enquiry. *Family Process, 48*(3), 319–331. https://doi.org/10.1111/j.1545-5300.2009.01285.x

de Shazer, S., Berg, I. K., Lipchik, E., Nunnally, E., Molnar, A., Gingerich, W. & Weiner-Davis, M. (1986). Brief therapy: Focused solution development. *Family Process, 25*(2), 207–221.

de Shazer, S., Dolan, Y., Korman, H., Trepper, T., McCollum, E. & Berg, I. K. (2021). *More than miracles* (2nd ed.). Routledge.

Epston, D., Lakusta, C. & Tomm, K. (2008). Haunting from the future: a congenial approach to parent-children conflict. In *Down Under and Up Over: Travels with narrative therapy* (pp. 97–112). AFT Pub.

Fiske, H. (2008). *Hope in action: solution-focused conversations about suicide.* New York: Routledge.

Fook, J. (2002). *Social work: Critical theory and practice.* London: Sage Publications.

Goffman, E. (1963). *Stigma: Notes on the management of spoiled identity.* Engelwood Cliffs, NJ: Prentice Hall.

Lipchik, E. (2002). *Beyond technique in solution-focused therapy: Working with emotions and the therapeutic relationship.* New York: The Guilford Press.

Reynolds, V. (2020). Trauma and resistance: 'hang time' and other innovative responses to oppression, violence and suffering. *Journal of Family Therapy.* doi:10.1111/1467-6427.12293

Reynolds, V. & White, J. (2012). Hate kills: A social justice response to "suicide". Retrieved from http://discoursesofprevention.com/post-symposium-activities/.

Todd, N. & Wade, A. (2004). Coming to terms with violence and resistance: From a language of effects to a language of responses. In T. Strong & D. Pare (eds), *Furthering talk: Advances in the discursive therapies.* New York: Kluwer Academic Plenum.

Turner, V. W. (1969). *The ritual process: Structure and anti-structure.* Aldine Publishing Company.

Turner, V. & Bruner, E. (Eds.). (1986). *The anthropology of experience.* Chicago: University of Illinois Press.

Van Gennep, A. (1960). *The rites of passage.* Chicago: University of Chicago Press.

Wade, A. (1997). Small acts of living: Everyday resistance to violence and other forms of oppression. *Contemporary Family Therapy, 19*(1), 23–39.

Wade, A. (2002). *From a language of effects to responses: Honouring our clients' resistance to violence.* New Therapist.

White, M. (2003). Narrative Practice and community assignments. *International Journal of Narrative Therapy and Community Work, 2003*(2), 17–55.

White, M. & Epston, D. (1990). *Narrative means to therapeutic ends.* New York: W.W. Norton.

Chapter 16

Navigating Children's Experience of Separation/ Divorce

One of the complex situations at the walk-in arises when the presenting concern involves separation and divorce, along with a custody and access dispute. Given that approximately four in every ten marriages in Canada experience divorce it makes sense that families seek assistance at the walk-in clinic when children struggle with the changes. For many reasons this presents complex circumstances that are important to take into consideration. Where many clinics will not meet with children when brought to the walk-in by one care giver amid separation or divorce, there are circumstances in which it is important to go forward with the single session conversation.[1]

Whether we meet with the children and caregivers or not, is a decision that is made after great consideration and discussion amongst the walk-in team. There are several aspects we want to consider that go into our decision-making. I will share a few of these here. From these considerations, emerge ideas about how to proceed and possible conversational territories to explore. For space reasons I will not share all those kinds of conversations here, but for now hopefully some of these ideas spark conversations at your clinics with your teams. These ideas have come out of many conversations with the excellent people I work with at my clinic as we have struggled with how to proceed. I want to thank them for their input and debate.

First, it is important to note many discourses shape the stories people hold about their experience of separation/divorce as they visit the walk-in clinic. Discourses shaping meaning about separation and divorce include but are not limited to legal, medical, psychiatric, psychological and personal. Any discourse influences what information and knowledge gets privileged and circulated. Dominant discourses shape people's meaning making and can serve to eclipse everyday know-how and common sense.

- Legal discourse invites an agenda in which people are seeking walk-in service for their child to "disclose" to a professional the detriment they suffer on visitations[2]. Caregivers may seek testimony that can be used to address

DOI: 10.4324/9781003431688-17

custody and access matters. They may find themselves referred to the walk-in by their lawyer for this reason.

- Medical discourse and the language of "the syndrome" such as parental alienation syndrome leaves out an appraisal of social context, the experiences of the child. It invites attempts to cure the affected child or ill parent. It's a gateway to psychiatric explanations.
- Psychiatric discourse can turn contextualized distress and "responses" (sadness, worry, navigating the new situation) into a disease, an aberration of the child. It lends permission to the drugging of children, especially when they are difficult with one parent or the other.
- Psychological discourse with an emphasis on linear causal thinking (Holzman, 2018) can influence a construction of parental responses and actions as purposefully destructive, manipulative, and vengeful. Those understandings can prove divisive leaving good intentions and parent preferences out of storylines.
- The personal discourses are shaped by all these discourses as well as past and recent experiences. They shape the meaning people make of the events related to divorce/separation. Gender stories, patriarchy, individualism can all play a part in meaning generation that furthers divide and conflict.

As a brief narrative therapist, understanding how discourses are related to what gets said and by who informs our practice. This helps us recognize and take into consideration the part they play in shaping the many stories of separation and divorce brought to the walk-in clinic. This informs how we proceed. I am not suggesting that any of these discourses are right or wrong. I am acknowledging that they shape the meaning making in different ways making visible different courses of action while marginalizing others. For my purposes some discourses may close down possibility while others grow possibility.

Another notion about discourses is that they support the power of some persons or groups, serving their agenda while leaving others to the sidelines. In the context of children's mental health, my priority is the child. Having an awareness of these discourses and how they shape meaning making, as well as how they may serve some individuals over others assists me to "stay within the child's best interests" rather than the interests of the people the discourse may be serving. Given this, we can make the most of a session by striving to stay connected to the child's world, their thoughts, feelings, and actions that inform their experiences and the know-how they generate and employ to navigate the transition.

Our pre-session questionnaire requires the person completing the form to indicate whether they are involved in a custody/access court dispute or not. It further requires them to acknowledge that they realize our organization does not get involved in custody/access disputes or provide assessments for legal action. Whether we meet with the child/caregiver or not at the walk-in clinic is determined by the Supervisor in consultation with lead therapist/team and is a situation-by-situation determination. The check box on the pre-session form highlights for us the need to have a specific conversation with the referent about the conditions under which we would consider meeting with their child and/or themselves. Some of the consideration and conditions are as follows:

- Would proceeding be in the best interest of the child?
- We hold the responsibility to ensure our contribution to the conversation resists escalating the situation and strives to provide a process supporting de-escalation.
- Both parents may be involved separately when it is deemed safe and fitting.
- We hold an influential yet de-centred position[3] seeking local knowledge—hopes wishes, preferences, skills, knowledges that can be brought forward to address the context of the youth's situation.
- We will not sponsor conversations that problematize or totalize a caregiver as we recognize the multi-storied aspects of life and relationships.
- We will not entertain conversations in which the referrer talks poorly of the other care giver.
- We view the child/youth as our primary concern and will meet with them to assist with finding ways to carry on amidst their life circumstances. However, we also recognize that discussing coping with the young person in the midst of adult discrepancy or conflict may unintentionally support living amongst ongoing conflict. Should we suspect emotional harm or physical harm might be occurring we will bring Child Protection Services into the conversation.
- We will not elicit conversations about the child's living arrangement "wishes" recognizing that those wishes involve a complexity of circumstances not easily heard in a time constrained conversation. Should the child bring this up, our conversation option is to inquire as to what that wish says about what the child values in all child/parent relationships and relationships in general.
- Our preference is to work in teams with a lead therapist and outsider witness or co-therapist to assist to inoculate against unintended alliances and pulls in the process.

Flags for NOT Proceeding

There are times when the team decides we will not proceed with meeting with the child due to circumstances that are like flags for us that therapy may cause difficulty. This is determined collectively and with tremendous consideration and scrutiny of the situation. Circumstances that have us consider not meeting with the child can include:

- If the parents have equal rights and one parent is not consenting.[4]
- There is ongoing exposure to violence, high conflict, or oppression. For instance, if the ex-partners are still living together through the transition of divorce be aware of the position the child may be in.
- The child is functioning well enough in life domains of school, relationships, community, family, and sleeping well enough.
- If the parent is seeking to have the child testify; that is wanting the therapist to elicit the child's feelings about the situation, visits to the partners home, or other arrangements.
- If the parent has been sent by a third party and is not sure why, (ex. a lawyer).
- If our meeting is to be kept secret from other parent, the other parent is unaware and/or in opposition to seeking therapeutic support on behalf of the child. This flag may be conditional depending on child protection service involvement.

Criteria for Proceeding

- If there is a safety concern related to the child. Ensuring safety trumps consent.
- If the child's daily living is suffering; that is if there is distress that is interfering with sleep, school, relationships with peers and family beyond what might be expected in these situations.
- If it seems apparent that the child is not amidst ongoing conflict.
- If the child is at an age and place where they can understand that their distress is in relation to the separation/divorce and understand the possible consequences of meeting.

Pre-meeting with a Care Giver

To determine whether to proceed or not very often the therapist will invite the care giver who brought the child into a pre-meeting to elicit further details to assist with making a decision. This conversation involves the following.

- Determine whose idea it was to come and what they were hoping for out of the conversation. If it is a third-party referral, ask what the referrer wanted by having the child and caregiver come to walk-in.
- Ask about the current custody agreement and if the other caregiver is aware of them coming to walk-in. We may seek confirmation of this through text or phone call at that time.
- Ask about the daily living of the child and if there is distress interfering with home, school, community, relationships, health.
- Note the pros and cons of proceeding.

- Highlight what conversations we will not have such as vilifying a caregiver, preferences for where to live, archiving the faults or bad experiences for the sake of getting evidence, getting the child to talk about the other parent.
- Highlight the kinds of conversations we will have such as conversations about responses and what they are founded on, coping, and ideas for adults.
- Reiterate non-involvement in custody/access proceedings.
- Provide resources when appropriate.
- Advise to return should daily living suffer to the point that the adult is struggling to assist.

Therapeutic Conversations Available to the Therapist?

With Referring Caregiver

- With either caregiver we can facilitate a "statement of position" conversation (White & Epston, 1990; White, 2007). This map may provide opportunity to begin an externalizing conversation objectifying the problem as "The Divorce", "Separation", "Conflict" etc.. It involves meeting with the lone parent/caregiver without the child and assisting them to explore the effects of the problem (the dispute) on the child/youth and how these effects may be incongruent with their intentions. They may gain a different look at the problem, adjust their position towards the problem, and employ different actions that are more congruent with their intentions. *When you and your ex-partner talk through the children like that, what do you suppose their experience is? When the children hear you talk poorly about your ex-partner what do you suppose it is like for them?*
- An excavation of "parent preferences" (Eron and Lund, 1996) can serve as a guide for future steps. *When you first held your child as a very small baby in your arms, what were your hopes for them? What sorts of skills did you want them to learn? How do you hope they describe you to their best friend? What stories do you want them to tell your future grandchildren about you and your parenting? How are you teaching them this through this dispute? What do you want your children to learn from you about how to navigate relationships through this dispute?*
- Excavation and development of "stories-in-the-making" related to parent preferences help to give these intentions more meaning. *You noted you were hoping to teach your child to be respectful, tell me a time that you were doing that? Where else does that teaching show up in your life? How are you doing that through this custody/access process?*
- Acquaint the caregiver with options available for proceeding with other complimentary services such as Women's Services, mediation, parent coordination, lawyers, parenting after separation and divorce workshop, etc.

- Bring child protection services into the conversation if there is emotional or physical harm suspected.
- Explore other possibilities. *What are your guesses about what caregivers who have divorced whose children have come through it in the healthiest way did to make that happen?*
- Co-creation of a take-away document archiving their preferences and plans that are congruent with their positive intentions. These documents serve as reminders of their intentions.

Conversations With the Youth

For youth who are out of the conflict but struggling to handle the circumstances of the separation/divorce, we can elicit their know-how learned in navigating parental conflict and separation. Drawing from Denborough (2010), we can be curious about:

- Ways they sought comfort, places they escaped to, relationships they turned to, actions they took, things they did, counter thoughts, feelings actions.
- What are the particular skills they have employed such as self-care skills, care for others, skills to navigate the circumstances. What is the foundation of those skills–values, beliefs they hold. Where/who did they learn that from?
- We can archive their advice to adults as to what children may need from adults in such situations.

These ideas can be brought into a take-away document in the form of a list or booklet to be shared with other youth, parents, care givers, or relatives.

Externalizing Conversations into Take-Away Documents

Often with youth I will invite them to craft a document that can be shared with the adults in their lives. This document archives the children's experiences and know-how in navigating parental separation.

- **Characterize and Name the Problem:** After some exploration of the situation, we can invite the youth to name the problem.
  - *What would you call this situation if you could give it a name?* I have heard the experience of separation /divorce called many things by children such as Living in a Tornado, The Split Up, The Big Bump.
- **Problem Resistance:** Explore with the youth what has sustained them given the Problem. This involves eliciting an account of how they have carried on at home, school, relationships? As Denborough would say, what sustains

them during hard times. Again, we can elicit an account of things they do and think to bring comfort, places and relationships they draw on like "stuffies".

- *Given "The Big Bump" how have you stopped things from getting worse for you?*
- *How do you not let sadness take you over?*
- *What do you do when the "Split Up" is bugging you?*
- *How do you handle missing a parent?*

- **Re-memberings:** Many children may be oriented to the more difficult times during a separation/divorce that serve to overshadow more preferred events. To elevate memories of better times and memories that may help support youth, I seek to elicit and archive those times.

  - *Do you have a favourite memory that you find warming or nice to keep?*
  - *If you were to give other children advice who were at the beginning of experiencing a Big Bump, what would you tell them is important to remember?* (About parents, about family, about themselves, about the situation)

- **Advice to Parents about Parenting:** Elicit the youth's advice for their parents about what they do that is helpful and not helpful to the youth. This is advice in relation to care giving the child and NOT advice to reconcile, or how one parent should treat the other.

  - *What do you need from your parents, grandparents that helps you to get used to things?*
  - *What do your parents do that you want them to keep doing?*

- **Document Construction and Distribution:** Seek permission to develop the take-away document along with the youth. Gain permission to share with other youth who may be up against a similar situation. Include blank pages at the back to record after-thoughts.

  - *Did you know there are other youth in similar situations experiencing their own Big Bumps?*
  - *Would you be willing to share this document with them by having it available in our waiting room?*
  - *Who would you like to share this document with, in your life? How many copies do you want?*
  - *Where would be a good place to keep this so that it is there when you need it?*
  - *When would be a good time to look it over and give it a read? Why, what difference will it make to you to look at it during those times?*

Closing

Separation, divorce and custody and access dispute situations present a realm of legal and relational complexity. This is especially present as children are brought to the walk-in for single session therapy. I have presented several considerations within this chapter for navigating this complexity while keeping the best interest of the child at the centre of the work. Working as a team to weigh options in these situations and for decision making helps to consider multiple perspectives and shore up a safe process for all, including the child and caregivers.

Notes

1 Agencies should have policy and procedure in place to guide who gets seen and when children don't get seen. It's important to follow your agency policy however hopefully that policy takes into consideration many of the scenarios that present at the walk-in clinic.
2 In these circumstances we encourage care givers to work with their local child protection services should they have concern that their child is at risk of harm. We try to prevent the single session from being a place to encourage children to disclose as follow-up to that testimony may contaminate their relationship to services for the future. That said, if we do receive information that a child may be at risk of harm, we bring child protection services into the conversation.
3 See White & Morgan, (2006) for an account of the influential yet de-centred position.
4 It is important to consider the consent and privacy legislation for your area. We endeavour to respect the rights of both parents. In our area, a youth at age 12 is able to be seen without a parent knowing or being involved.

References

Denborough, D. (2010). To come to reasonable terms with one's own history: Children, parents and mental health. *Context,* April, 63–67.

Eron, J. B. & Lund, T. W. (1996). *Narrative solutions in brief therapy.* New York: Guilford Press.

Holzman, L. (2018). *The overweight brain: How our obsession with knowing keeps us from getting smart enough to make a Better World.* East Side Institute Press.

White, M. (2007). *Maps of narrative practice.* New York: W.W. Norton.

White, M. & Epston, D. (1990). *Narrative means to therapeutic ends.* New York: W.W. Norton.

White, M. & Morgan, A. (2006). *Narrative therapy with children and their families.* Adelaide, South Australia: Dulwich Centre Publications.

Chapter 17

Developing Concepts for Living

Narrative practice has always drawn from a diverse field of ideas well outside traditional psychology. In his later writings, Michael White (2006, 2007, 2011) referenced the work of Russian Psychologist Lev Vygotsky (1978, 1987) whose work focused on child development. A key Vygotskian (1978) understanding emphasizes that learning is an achievement through social collaboration rather than an independent effort. Within this collaboration, Vygotsky described a learning zone called the zone of proximal development wherein learning is social and incremental. This zone is the space between what is known and what is possible to know and can only be traversed when it is broken down into manageable tasks or steps. These tasks provide a scaffold for children's development of concepts which assist them to gradually move from collaborative to independent performance.

With these Vygotskian principles as a lens through which to view narrative practice, Michael came to talk about his therapeutic conversations as assisting people to distance from the known and familiar of their lives. Therapeutic conversations assist people across the zone of proximal development towards what is possible to know and do as concepts are co-developed that assist people to navigate life. He saw the maps of narrative therapy and the questions within the maps as providing the scaffolding for this incremental movement leading to the development of those concepts that would prove useful to people when they return to their daily living. Through concept development, people could begin to more independently direct their lives and experience personal agency.

Informed by these ideas, White crafted the scaffolding conversations map (2007, 2011). This map revises his maps one and two, situating them as a scaffold to move across the zone of proximal development. It was proposed that in this space, through the linking of experiences (re-authoring), concepts were developed. In an interesting research study, Heather Ramey (2010) investigated the use of narrative maps in single session therapy conversations. She was able to demonstrate, as Michael suspected, the development of concept formation in single session therapy using the scaffolding conversations map.

DOI: 10.4324/9781003431688-18

Movement through the zone of proximal development from the known and familiar towards what's possible to know and do overlays very well onto our rites of passage metaphor. The liminal space within the rite of passage represents the zone of proximal development (Duvall & Berés, 2011) that can be crossed through social collaboration with a senior partner, that being the therapist. For single session therapy, we can begin to define a useful session as one in which the participant experiences any movement from the known and familiar. That movement can be large or quite small and anywhere in between. I'll elaborate on our measure of a useful single session further in Chapter 18. For our purpose in this chapter, the idea of concept development assists us to think about our conversations differently. The single session conversation becomes a venue within which concepts can be co-developed and re-contextualize into everyday life. It is a process that aligns with the idea that practice happens after the therapy encounter within people's everyday life. Concepts provide the tools with which to practice.

Definition of a Concept

A concept is defined as, "Something conceived in the mind: thought, notion, an abstract or generic idea generalized from particular instances" (Stein, 1980 p. 278). As ideas that give meaning to our world, they are based upon a person's own previous experiences. Concepts help to reduce the complexity of the world and assist us to respond to it efficiently. We navigate life with many important concepts such as friendship, death, celebration, strengths, loneliness, and so on. Concepts, in the therapeutic context, are developed frequently whether it's the notion of a diagnosis, a strength, resilience, or transference.

Each of these concepts serves to umbrella a series of experiences in the form of thoughts, feelings, and actions that have been connected and associated. In this associating and connecting, other actions, thoughts, and feelings become excluded as they do not relate or fit the theme of the association. As these associations are formed, concepts are developed that bring the complexity of the associations and the complexity of life into a focus.

Think, for example, about the concept of friendship. As you grew, through various social experiences you came to sort out which relationships qualified as a friendship, and which did not. The name "friendship" came to be applied to those that fit the bill so to speak. This concept of friendship emerged from many experiences. Over time, through interactions you came to define friendship as meeting specific thoughts about people, feelings towards them, and connected actions such as doing fun things together. As this concept evolved from a preconcept to a full concept, it now assists you to discern that not everyone you encounter is a friend. You no longer need your caregivers to do this for you, to sort who to spend time with and who not to. As you have adopted the concept, you can now act independently on your relationships, sorting and cultivating them. The concept of friendship now brings all the complexity of the past thoughts, feelings, and actions into a simplified notion making life easier.

Although concepts reduce the complexity of life, they do not necessarily assist people in preferred ways in the context of therapy. Some concepts can have the effect of freezing people's life journey and identity. These kinds of concepts often relate to their perceived deficits, and negative identity conclusions, which have them blinded to possible skills and abilities that could make new initiatives possible.

Concepts for Living

My preference is to move the conversation towards the naming and development of what I refer to as "concepts for living". Concepts for living are those concepts mutually developed through the linking of expressions of thoughts, feelings, and actions across time that allow people to live life in harmony with their values, hopes, wishes, and preferences. It is in the development of concepts for living that people can begin to make plans and have ideas about which next steps in their life may be possible and preferred.

The development of concepts for living begins by facilitating an experience or establishing mutual attention towards a preferred experience. That selected experience most often builds off the person's past experience or is in relation to their own interests. With mutual attention to the experience, I invite the person to attach a name to assist with concept formation. This is congruent with White's (2007) first level[1] of the distancing conversations map. I may offer suggestions, but the name needs to be agreed upon by the participant. Through the use of questions, we then seek other experiences including thoughts, feelings and actions that fit with the developing concept, inviting the participant to link and connect these. These questions are, in part, reflected in levels two through four of White's map canvasing effects on life and relationships, feelings about themselves, realizations and learnings, and reflections on what is made possible. Lastly, and as an important part of the single session therapy map, we co-develop plans for when they leave, how they will navigate with the evolving concept. I document their knowledge so that it can be revisited and shared with others with permission. The use of play often helps in the exploration of concepts and the word/meaning connection.

Experiential Activities

Gadamer (in Grondin, 2002) notes the indication that a concept is understood and useful to someone if it's demonstrated cognitively (I get it), linguistically (I can put it into words), and practically (I can apply it). This highlights the importance of performance through experiential activities. Activities assist with concept development and the enactment of the preferred story-in-the-making.

I use several multi-modal play-based activities to assist with concept development with children and their caregivers in a single session of therapy. These activities allow for the development of or further development of concepts that assist children and their families to navigate their predicaments following our time together. I think about the project within the single session to facilitate preferred experience and to assist the child to enact the preferred story-in-the-making along with the caregiver. The skills the caregivers are seeking will take practice and growth. It will be a work in progress, so I use the session to provide a venue for the child to show that they have the beginnings of the concept/skill and then co-create the plan to grow the concept/skill in context.

For instance, when meeting children who have suffered early developmental trauma they can be seen as quite busy, energetic, and they may experience emotional responses intensely, at times becoming overwhelmed by frustration, anger, or sadness. Caregivers may be experiencing a sense of failure and loss for how to continue on with their child. Some children arrive labelled as conduct disordered or oppositional defiant, reflecting their struggle to comply with instruction or accept being told "no" by the adults in their life. The project, most often outlined by the caregiver, is for their child to "regulate their emotions" as the concept of dis-regulation has been applied. They want the child to listen better or accept their instruction more quickly. While these are sensible wishes, they represent a project that is likely beyond achievable in the time available.

To look at trying to accomplish the broader project in one conversation will certainly be met with a sense of discouragement and futility. However, what is possible is to begin to co-develop concepts for living that when taken home and practiced, assist the youth and family to navigate their circumstances. I find using fun engaging activities helps with concept development providing experiences to build from. Understanding our time together as a definitional ceremony allows a space in which, together, we can play or preform more preferred ways of being in the world away from the constraint of problem solving.

Balance Boards

One young person I met with took to leaping from couch to chair in our meeting space, back and forth and free of redirection. It looked fun, so I could understand the attraction but the adult in me was worried for their safety as each leap became more daring. Between the acrobatics they also proceeded to snap the leaves of the tropical plants in the room one by one. I could just imagine our caretakers of these plants wincing from afar with each snap.

I try to meet children in their world and use the material they bring to these conversations be it what they say or what they do. Many children will bring a favourite toy with them which provides a helpful entry point into our work together. In this moment, I was thinking about the metaphor of a rushing river. The idea is, if you fall into a rushing river you don't swim against the current as you'll likely quickly tire and drown. Rather, the most helpful course of action is to swim with the current but work your way towards shore as you go. Similarly, Erikson's notion of utilization (Haley, 1993) also works well in these situations. The idea is to use whatever the person brings to the process in a useful way. To "swim with" the child's interest and to help the plants survive, I invited him to jump a few more times from one couch to the other. He was quite skilled at this, but I spotted him to shore up the safety.

Now that I had canvassed his cooperation, to engage this young person further but also to facilitate the development of a concept for living, I introduced the family to the balance boards. I had learned about balance boards from colleague with an interest in body work. These are specifically constructed boards with a crescent shaped bottom to allow them to teeter tauter. The use of balance boards facilitates the experience of internally regulating a turbulent external environment. I enticed the youth with a challenge noting, "I bet you can't balance on this board more than 30 seconds". He accepted my challenge and exceeded it with ease. Playfully, I introduced increasingly difficult challenges. Can you do that with your eyes closed? Can you balance on one foot? Can you touch your toes? With each step his concentration and control of himself grew. Finally, I stated, "Wow I think you're ready to level up"; a video game metaphor that he related well to. I then proceeded to throw soft objects to be caught while balancing. At times, you can try juggling together which is a great way to teach breathing, the concept of concentration, and turn taking.

Now experiencing a sense of success and competence he decided he needed to stack two boards on top of one another igniting the worry of the adults in the room. He certainly could fall in this challenge however it provided opportunity for us to inject the concept of "safety" into the experience. Prompting the caregivers to join in, we began to lay pillows around the youth while narrating how things were getting a bit unsafe and we were feeling worried so we wanted to make the situation *safer* so *we* could relax. The emphasis was on the connection to safety and its help to the adults as not to canvas push back if it was directed at making it safer for the child. In this process the youth experienced a moment in which the adults in his life provided safety. This was very different from the experience he had of adults prior to being taken to a place of safety by child protection services. This was a piece of the story-in-the-making informing the theme that there are safe responsive adults in the world at the same time orienting the child's attention to safety in general.

Our questions are important in these scenarios. As the child was balancing, I was curious, asking:

- How are you doing that? [Eliciting their skill, ability, and implying personal agency.]
- How are you able to go so long?
- Did you have to change your breathing? [Linking to the physical.]

- What are you thinking to yourself? [Linking to thoughts.]
- What happens if you put your arms out or to the side is it easier or harder?
- What about if you close your eyes? What difference does that make?
- What do you call that skill you are using? [Naming the concept linked to thoughts, feelings, actions.] "My calmness."
- If 10/10 is the superpower of calmness and 1 is the opposite, how calm do you have yourself right now? How much calmer can you go?
- How are you calming yourself like that?
- If 10/10 is super safe and 1 is the opposite, how safe were you before the pillows were put in place? How safe are you now that they are in place? What other ideas do you have to make this even safer?
- What are you learning about yourself? [Drawing out realizations and learnings.]
- To the caregiver, "Did you know your child had this ability? What's it like to see them meet this challenge and find their calmness?"

These questions assist in concept development, languaging into existence the child's skills of calming, self-control, and regulation. In answering, the child is oriented to their competency and comes to experience their ability to direct themselves and their life. While these emerging skills may not be highly advanced at this stage, their identification and practice set the scene for future practice and use of the concept of "calmness" in everyday life. To grow the concepts, I invite families to "play this game" at home, simply balancing on one foot or the other inviting practice in the real world. Children are invited to teach their caregiver about their skills and abilities.

Remote Controls

I came across the remote-control activity some years ago and adapted it for the use in single session therapy to facilitate concept development related to self-control, focus, and concentration. Most families can relate to and understand the function of a remote control for a television or video game console that allows them to control the device, change the channel, adjust the volume, etc.

First, I elicit their willingness to play a game and I explain why I'm introducing it.

I wonder if you would like to play a game as a fun way to practice some of the skills you are hoping to teach your child and for you to show off the skills you already have? [To the child] I bet your caregiver doesn't realize how skilled you are at some of this. Maybe you are shy and don't like to show off these skills, or maybe you forget them sometimes, so I hope we can play this game to learn some of these from you.

We then break out the craft supplies and I walk them through creating remote control devices. We wrap a small box with paper, and I prompt them to think about what buttons they would like to include such as play, fast-forward, rewind, slow motion, etc. I may ask, "What button do you think is the most important for your family? What other buttons should we include: I need a hug, I need space, wait your turn, listen, etc.?" Using stickers and labels, each family member places their buttons and crafts a remote. Then the fun begins.

Starting with the child, I ask them to test out the remote with me. Pointing the remote at them, I test the volume first. I say, "Okay I'm turning volume down." Most times the youth quiets their voice to a whisper. I then volume up to a very loud level which is easily matched. Once again, I volume down to an acceptable level for indoors. We then proceed to test the movement buttons. Asking them to run on the spot or in a circle depending how much space we have, I press and narrate "play" then "fast forward". Once in fast-forward, I then test the pause button as a means to challenge the youth with the most difficult circumstance. Once paused, I wait and wait and wait until just before I sense they can't hold it any longer. I then resume working through "rewind", "slow motion" (my favourite) and finally back to "play". As the child follows along, I confirm, "Okay this remote is working". We then proceed to take turns using the remotes to direct each other. The child directs the caregiver then the caregiver directs the child with the spirit of fun and play.

Once again, our questions during this process are important to highlight the ability of the child to direct their actions and choices, for concept development, for inviting a name for the skill they are employing, and to assist the skill to move from pre-concept to a fuller concept. The use of "how" questions and by inviting them to mentor us in the practice elicits the child's ability to direct their actions and choices. I reference back to when the child was able to pause so long. How did you manage to pause like that? Again, inviting the child to give a name to the skill is an important step in concept development. Is that a skill or ability you were using? What do you call that skill? At times I editorialize, "Is that your concentration, self-control, or calmness?" Together, we are languaging into existence the concept for living. Lastly, questions that assist the movement from pre-concept to fuller concept invite the linking of an action to thoughts, feelings and other actions.

Expanding the process, it's important to invite participants to contextualize the skill into the future through performance. Again, using our questions we enter into speculation and practice. When would it be most important for this skill to show up at home? Okay, can we act this out? First, let's act out when you don't use the skill. We then proceed to assign roles, structure the scene, and "action" is called. It's then time to generalize the emerging concept. Okay, now let's replay the scene but this time use your skill of concentration and let's see how things go. "Action" is once again called, and the scene begins with noticeable differences. At times, pauses are called to rework the scene but with a continued spirit of humour and fun. The youth is consulted often for their direction and fine-tuning. What should the adults do here? What would you do next? Okay, should we try it that way? Finally, the action plan is co-created outlining when to further practice the developed concept, outlining what would be signs of improvement, and when might they need to return to the walk-in for fine-tuning the plan[2].

Life Club Rules for Relationships

There are many means by which people can lose their way in relationships. Often children are brought to the walk-in struggling with relationships in their lives. These struggles have come about through breaches in those relationships in some way. It may be through the experience of bullying. In those circumstances they find themselves vulnerable to a sense of isolation and negative conclusions about themselves shaped by the relationship trespasses.

Sometimes children are brought by a non-parental relative with whom they reside. The alternate living arrangement has come about as the child's parent has restricted access by Child Protective Services due to safety concerns. Many of these children had experienced distressing early childhood experiences during their time with the parent. When contact in the form of phone calls or visits are a means to re-establish relationship with the biological parent, it can be difficult for children. They struggle to navigate these arrangements put in place by the adults/authorities. The children are brought to the walk-in by the custodial caregiver out of concern that they are experiencing nightmares, sadness, withdrawal from activities, fear and frustrations related to these often-mandated circumstances.

Other times, I meet people who have experienced abuse in relationships. They have endured mistreatment, experienced multiple relationships with abuse and have lost their way in a current relationship. For them, it can be difficult to know their relationship preferences and they may present distress that they don't necessarily connect to the past mistreatment.

In addressing these relationship stories and to facilitate concept development it has been useful to introduce the "club of life" metaphor (White, 1997). This metaphor likens one's life to a club consisting of various memberships. These members and their membership can be made visible and discussed. People in one's life club can be allocated different memberships depending on their actions. As in any club, perhaps some memberships are elevated whereas others are downgraded, suspended, or cancelled.

Inviting children, youth, and adults to reflect on the relationships in their life club introduces important concepts such as the notion that they can revise relationships and have a say about them. We can figure out with them which voices have credibility and can be listened to on matters of identity. Together, we can discern those who lack credibility and identify a membership that needs revising if needed. Alternatively, new members can be selected, recruited, and auditioned.

In these matters the intention is to create space for the person's relationship preferences to be made visible and responded to. I am striving to learn from them what's important to them in relationships and support a sense that they can shape the relationships in their life. Further, as members are consulted about identity the intention is to shore up preferred understandings of identity.

In situations specific to renewing relations with a parent, the child's wishes are often in the background, overshadowed by the good intentions of adults. In these situations, it is important to me not to totalize a parent as harmful but rather to recognize people are multi-storied and to leave future relationship options open. A parent can make changes in their life. A child can experience a parent who uses abuse in loving or caring ways as well. I want them to share their ideas about how the relationship should be; their relationship preferences.

Lastly, I want to assist people to create a document that archives their ideas which can be shared and serve as a guide for relationships. It can be a means to hold adults accountable to doing relationships safely. It can assist adults not to lose their way in relationships. It can assist children to see they are not alone in the face of bullying.

Step 1: Introduce the "Life Club" metaphor:
The first step is to introduce the "Life Club" metaphor (White, 1997):

> Would it be okay if I share with you an idea I came across about relationships? This is how we draw the different relationships in our life (I draw circles on a piece of paper similar to a target and place the person's name at the very centre). It's called My Life Club. In the centre we put you and then these circles are the different memberships in your club. There are inner circle memberships; the people you are closest to and who follow the rules you set for your club. Then there are other members that may be new to the club or sometimes follow the rules. These might be friends, classmates, etc. Then on the outer edges are the people seeking membership in your club.

Step 2: Learn about and record Life Club rules:
To draw out relationship preferences as well as preferred experiences of relationships, I invite participants to share the rules or guidelines to be a member of their club.

> Before we place relationships in your club, let's get down some of the rules that they have to follow in order to be part of it. For instance, what are your ideas about how people should treat each other? What are your ideas about how the phone calls should go? What shouldn't happen or be allowed? What are your rules for adults? Where or when did you learn that that would be a

good Life Club rule? Who did you learn that from or with? What difference does it make to you when you are with people following that rule?

I hear many expressions of relationship preferences and rules. Melody, age 7, was brought to the walk-in by her grandmother as she was having nightmares and upset tummy. Her child protection worker had recently reinstated phone calls between Melody and her biological mother. Previous contact had been prohibited due to her mother's volatile moods and the hurtful things she would say to Melody. As part of Melody's club rules, she was clear that to be in her club:

* Don't talk about the old days on the phone.
* No yelling at me.
* Talk about things I like.

Rachel a teenager navigating a family split shared her Rules to Navigate the Sea of Life:

* Keep it to yourself, meaning don't talk badly about other family members.
* Don't bring up stuff that gets too personal such as pressuring about where to live.
* Remember the people that you love are more important than ANYTHING else.

Step 3: Invite to list and place relationships in the club and reflect:

Alright, so we have some important club rules here, now who would you list in your inner circle; the relationships most important, those who meet your requirements, or that you are closest to? Who do you enjoy but maybe aren't as close to as these other people? Who would you place in your club but more on the outside; perhaps someone who follows some of the rules but not all of them, perhaps someone you don't see often but appreciates you and you them? Are there any pets that make it into the club? How come you would place them there? What do they do that you like or don't care for? When is it good to get some distance from them or draw them closer?

Step 4: Invite to make meaning of the Life Club:
It's in the reflexive moments that people come up with the next steps in life. Once the rules are stated and members situated, I invite the participant to step back to take a look at their club. Within this different vantage point, I ask questions to assist them to make sense of this exercise and what it means to them.

Did you know you had this many people in your Life Club? What is it like to know you have this many people? What difference will it make when you leave here to know you have this many in your club? If I could talk to the people at the centre of your club what is your guess about what they would say to me, they appreciate about you? What might they tell me they like about your friendship? Who do you see as a trustworthy voice or a credible reference about you?

These kinds of conversations support the development of concepts related to positive and preferred identity conclusions, preferred relationship markers, and help to restore a sense of personal agency in relationships. When followed-up with our phase three questions, people will share their ideas about how these concepts can and will shape their future interactions and understandings in useful ways.

This chapter has placed an emphasis on the idea of developing concepts for living in single session therapy. Through linking thoughts, feelings, and actions across time, drawing from people's lived experiences, concepts can be highlighted, practiced, and generalized into the receiving context of people's lives.

Notes

1 For a detailed account of White's Scaffolding Conversations Map see the chapters, *Scaffolding Conversations in Maps of Narrative Practice* p. 263–290, as well as *Scaffolding a Therapeutic Conversation in Masters of Narrative and Collaborative Therapies* p. 121–170.
2 Often, I'll invite caregivers to craft a specific 'Therapeutic Parenting Plan' that includes their ideas about how to continue to practice the concept we began forging in the single session. These plans come about after discussion of how caregivers have been able to teach some skills to their child already. There are always skills to reference. Then we add in what to apply to teaching the concept that is developing. The concept of a 'therapeutic' parenting plan also seems useful positioning caregivers as co-therapists, able to facilitate the learning.

References

Duvall, J. & Béres, L. (2011). *Innovations in narrative therapy: Connecting practice, training, and research.* New York: W. W. Norton.
Grondin, J. (2002). Gadamer's basic understanding of understanding. In R. Dostal (Ed.), *The Cambridge companion to Gadamer* (pp. 36–51). Cambridge University Press.
Haley, J. (1993). *Uncommon therapy: The psychiatric techniques of Milton H. Erickson, M.D.* W. W. Norton.
Ramey, H.L., Young, K. & Tarulli, D. (2010). Scaffolding and concept formation in narrative therapy: A qualitative research report. *Journal of Systemic Therapies, 29*, 74–91.
Stein, J. (Ed.). (1980). *The Random House College Dictionary* (Revised Edition). Random House Inc.
Vygotsky, L.S. (1978). *Mind in society: The development of higher psychological processes.* Harvard University Press.

Vygotsky, L.S. (1987). *The collected works of L.S. Vygotsky* (R.W. Rieber & A. S. Carton, Eds.). Plenum Press.

Vygotsky, L.S., Rieber, R.W. & Carton, A.S. (1987). *The collected works of L. S. Vygotsky*, Vol. 1: Problems of general psychology.

White, M. (1997). Re-membering. In M. White *Narratives of therapists lives.* Adelaide: Dulwich Centre Publications.

White, M. (2007). *Maps of narrative practice*. New York: W.W. Norton.

White, M. (2011). *Narrative practice: Continuing the conversations*. New York: W.W. Norton.

White, M. & Morgan A. (2006). *Narrative therapy with children and their families.* Adelaide: Dulwich Centre Publications.

Chapter 18

Quality Assurance in Single Session Therapy

Originally, the emergence of walk-in or quick access therapy clinics spawn from concern over long wait lists for mental health service. Organizations were looking for a means to get services to the people as soon as possible and to clear away the traditions of long assessment and paperwork that, in part, created barriers to service. The spirit of the walk-in clinic and single session therapy was to provide quick access, to get the product to the people in their time of need. The intention was to facilitate a useful, complete therapy encounter that assists people to address their most pressing concern. This was a wonderful and caring intention. How can we be there for people when they need us?

Increasingly, I have become concerned about where the practice is headed. As SST grew in popularity, we have seen many authorities with diverse interests begin to shape the landscape of service further. Some agencies have defined their brand of SST and invite the use of very diverse models of therapy in a single encounter. That is not what I advocate for. Some approaches benefit most from ongoing work where ideas and suggestions can be monitored, followed up about, and further shaped. Still, other approaches that obscure personal agency or medicalize distress are not meant for this context.

Several agencies in Ontario are using their walk-in as the front door to ongoing service (Catalina, 2022). For most, I imagine this was a move to position services earlier in the path or continuum of service. Yet again, it is not a practice I would advocate for. Walk-in as a front door changes the context of the conversation. The focus risks becoming about deciding on my next service fit and timing rather than working to generate possibility within the assumption that this single conversation may be all that is needed. Walk-in single session therapy as access or intake is a very different kind of conversation than we have been exploring together.

An even more alarming development has been a push to implement standardized tools pre and post session. These tools are shaped by a diagnostic backdrop, and risk contaminating the work through influencing the meaning people make of their experiences prior to beginning their session. They direct attention to

DOI: 10.4324/9781003431688-19

problematic circumstances and consequently away from competence and the material that proves most useful to people in making changes.

For instance, some agencies have advocated for and even put into use a modified inter-RAI screener. The inter-RAI is a device to assess, respond to, and monitor mental health status and needs of vulnerable populations of children and youth. As well intentioned as they may be, to me this is a flawed approach to SST and not in harmony with our brief narrative practice intentions. Again, the context of walk-in/quick access therapy was to remove these kinds of barriers and influences.

This is not to say that I am against a pre/post tool but to rather note that I have not come across one that is a fit for our purposes. There are possibilities. Quantitative scaling for example provides self-anchored scales for people to situate their experiences and are easily understood by children and youth. This is a part of contemporary collaborative, competency-based, person-centred approaches. We can collaborate with participants about risk and safety and engage in conversations that generate possibility rather than document decontextualized problems. In this way we would embrace what White (2011) refers to as ethics of accountability within the screening/assessment process where we are accountable to what we do and the consequences of those interactions on the people that consult to us. In the end, any future tool needs "participatory co-design with diverse stakeholders to ensure equitable implementation" (Sukhara J., personal communication).

In response to these sorts of influences, in 2013 I crafted a post session feedback tool.[1] I was worried about one being mandated by funders that would not be compatible with our brief narrative, postmodern informed practice. At the time, walk-in clinics were fast growing throughout Ontario, so it was also very important to develop outcome and quality assurance measures relevant to time-constrained single session service delivery models.

Typical psychotherapy outcome measures take an extended view to measure the short and long-term goals of a program. Given the single session nature of walk-in clinics, often there is not the luxury of time, continued contact, or staffing to elicit data other than immediately following the session. Longer-term outcome studies, when employed at walk-in clinics, are often achieved through funding grants, volunteer services, or as funded research studies. For most children's mental health clinics, similar to the one at which I work, the use of three and six month, or one year outcome evaluations of the walk-in session are not a possibility. There is a "…lack of resources available for quality assurance and evaluation to measure and monitor program effectiveness and outcomes" (Children's Mental Health Ontario, 2013, p. 6). Base funding does not cover such initiatives and it is challenging to organize the necessary teams to apply for research funding. While many clinics utilize immediate post-session questioning to focus on determining whether people found the session helpful or had experiences such as friendly staff or easy access, these measures tell us little about people's experience of the conversation itself (quality assurance) and contribute little to the skill development of the therapist.

In considering outcomes, admittedly there's no perfect therapy. Data suggesting positive outcomes does not mean we are exempt from facilitating a process that has been hazardous, flawed, or incongruent with our intentions. This invites important discussion about ethics and practice ethics. As discussed in Chapter 2, we embrace relational ethics as a guide that brings attention to how we do what we do and the possible effects. The process is as important as the outcome.

Process as Outcome

In review of post-session SST data at our clinic, people don't comment things like "Wow, Scot's clinical wizardry blew me away" or "That externalizing was so Michel White like." They do comment things like "I was greeted with a smile the minute I walked in," "They nourished me physically (we always have snacks available) and mentally", and "I felt safe, listened to, and understood where I'm coming from". These sorts of comments caught my attention, so I started sorting and grouping over five years of post-session data into what I call PART(s)[2] of single session therapy; Process, Actions, Resources, and Thinking. Results show that people comment over 30% of the time about their experience of the session, that is about the process. Interestingly, just under 40% comment on leaving with new strategies (Actions) and almost 30% comment on how they are seeing themselves or their situation differently (Thinking). A very small percentage comment on the usefulness of receiving service resources. For me, this highlights the importance of attention to how we do what we do, the process of the single session.

The process of a therapeutic encounter "…includes everything that transpires between and within the participants when they are actually or virtually in each other's presence" (Orlinsky, Ronnestad, & Willutzki, 2004, p. 311). Narrative practice places an emphasis on attention to the process of the therapy itself (how we do what we do together and the possible effects of what we do) alongside the outcomes of the therapeutic encounter (the usefulness of what we do together). The single session timed constrained context of a walk-in clinic places great responsibility on the therapist to respect the relational ethics of narrative therapy given there often are not opportunities to address mishaps in future contacts or follow-up.

Orlinsky et al. (2004) highlight the "…interrelations of various process facets with one another and ultimately with outcome" (p. 320). This notion, relating process to outcome, is relevant to quality assurance and outcome measures for single session therapy encounters. Resisting a process/outcome distinction and considering the time constraint of brief narrative single session therapy, how the person consulting us experiences the conversation provides the foundation for, and is intimately connected to, the outcome of the session. A measure of a single session is most useful when it provides information about the person's experience of the process as that is what's indicative of outcome in such time constrained circumstances.

Therapist Accountability and Learning

As I have said, measures are not neutral but rather have an effect not only on the participants of SST, but just as mush on the therapists themselves. Madsen furthers this point noting, "…what we attempt to measure and how we attempt to measure it have effects on clients, workers, and therapeutic relationships" (Madsen, 2007, p. 345). He continues noting, "… such questions subtly organize our interactions with families" (p.350). The questions we ask in a post-session questionnaire together with the responses to those questions will shape the future practices of the therapist. They serve to orient the therapist to the execution of certain micro-skills and ways of practicing that are preferred or in harmony with specific practice ethics. For instance, a post session question eliciting the participants rating of their experience of being asked about their skills and abilities, orients the therapist to be sure this is part of their practice. In this respect, post session questionnaires provide a learning tool for the therapist alongside data related to quality and outcome. The therapist can study the feedback as comment on their execution of the process assisting them to learn from each encounter.

Post-Session Questionnaires

The evolution of post-session questionnaires has been well influenced by the common factors movement that seeks to define what works in therapy (Duncan, Miller, Wampold & Hubble, 2010). Practitioners, researchers, and scholars such as Scott Miller (2003), Barry Duncan (2012), Lynn Johnson (1995), and Michael Lambert (2010) have advocated for and developed various measures seeking feedback from participants related to their experience of the process of therapy and outcomes. Specifically, over the past several decades (Duncan, Miller & Sparks, 2004; Duncan & Miller, 2000) advocate for the use of the Outcome Rating Scale (ORS) and the Session Rating Scale (SRS), two very brief instruments for monitoring the process and outcome of therapy. They take an empirically based, quantitative approach utilizing post-session questioning to elicit information from participants to shape therapist practices in future sessions.

Within this movement, I have been specifically drawn to Lynn Johnson's session rating scale (1995). This paper document elicits participant ratings along a continuum of criteria including experience of acceptance, liking/positive regard, understanding, therapist honesty and sincerity, agreement on goals, agreement on tasks, smoothness of the session, depth, helpful/usefulness and lastly hope (Duncan & Miller, 2000, p. 239).

These elements orient us to pay attention to how the person may have experienced the process of the session and practices employed by the therapist. The focus on the person's experience of the therapy and how that information could not only shape the therapy but also assist therapists in adjusting their practice opens important possibilities for assessing brief narrative single session therapy. Similar, post-session rating based on a continuum has also been used in the Session Evaluation Questionnaire (SEQ) by William Stiles (2002), designed to measure post-session the value and comfort of a session of psychotherapy.

Madsen in reviewing measures in collaborative therapy (Madsen, 2007 p. 350.), proposes several questions eliciting participants' input that align more closely with my brief narrative practice intentions than the Johnson Session Rating Scale (SRS) elements and phrasing. He proposes questions seeking feedback about therapists' efforts to understand the uniqueness of the person's life and what was the extent to which their "...abilities, skills and wisdom were acknowledged" (p. 350). Further, questions seek to learn to what extent participants felt they were active participants in the work, asking about their experience of a collaborative process.

The SSIFT

Adapting a post-session rating format (Duncan et al., 2000, 2004; Stiles, 2002), process questioning (Johnson, 1994), and expanding upon Madsen's languaging, I have crafted the Single Session Impressions and Feedback Tool (SSIFT)©, a tool to elicit process/outcome information about brief narrative walk-in clinic conversations (see Appendix 4). As an acronym, the SSIFT lives up to its name assisting us to sort through the complexity of a single session conversation to elicit the participants' experiences. This is a post-session questionnaire that looks at outcome as intimately linked to and influenced by process. The questionnaire seeks the perspective of participants, aged 11 and older, immediately following the session and is administered by the walk-in clinic receptionist. The SSIFT includes eight contrasting items along a 7-point scale. One supplement question requires a written response.

The questionnaire is not intended to be a traditional research tool subject to multiple trials seeking reliability or validity for strict adherence in employment by agencies and private practitioners to justify outcomes to funders and policy makers. My project is much more of a "collaborative ethnographic" (Lassiter, 2005) study. In part, the aim is to generate a cultural understanding of the session. I am seeking the "insider's point of view" and an understanding of the experiences generated in the culture of brief narrative single session therapy. What emerges are comments on categories of practice. The participants' experience of the conversation comes more available for consideration by the therapist. This subjective sharing then holds the therapist accountable for the part they play in that ethnography.

Questionnaire Criteria

There are many criteria that could be examined in a questionnaire, however, I want to examine those that are in line with my brief narrative practice, and that will assist me in my skill development, as well as hold me accountable to my practice ethics. Johnson's criteria included in the Session Rating Scale (1994) are items "...known to be associated with effective clinical work" (Duncan & Miller, 2000). This is an important consideration as our brief narrative approach looks to be effective, efficient, and in harmony with our relational ethics. The following are criteria suggestions along those lines.

Focus

As outlined in Chapter 5, brief narrative therapy is not a therapy in which goals are developed and pursued throughout the conversation as in other traditions of therapy. As a brief narrative conversation is a re-authoring conversation, or a conversation that provides the opportunity for people to more richly describe some of their skills for living and knowledges of life connected to alternate stories, the notion of "exploring conversational territory" (White, 2007) is a better fit. However, to remain efficient, together with the participants I need to share in outlining the conversational territory for the limited time we have together. Early in the conversation we discuss what would be most important to talk about to ensure the conversation remains as relevant as possible to the people consulting me.

Asking participants to rate "Focus" as a priority on the questionnaire holds the therapist to a practice ethic to ensure the conversation has remained relevant to the person consulting to us. We can ask people to discern on a continuum their experience asking if the conversation addressed what they wanted to talk about the most or seemed more focused on what the therapist wanted to discuss (Duncan et al., 2000). This is different from agreement on goals developed. Focus brings coherence to the conversation but allows for the conversation to explore many kinds of entry points to "stories-in-the-making".

Interest

I ask participants to provide a rating discerning between "The conversation caught and held my interest" and "The conversation interested me very little". This consideration of "interest" is not in the sense of entertainment value but rather a comment on questioning skills. I understand interest caught and held as a reflection of the therapists' ability to ask the kinds of questions that have people becoming curious about and interested in the unfolding meanings and understandings about their life and identity.

Hancock and Epston (2008) emphasize the learned craft and art of narrative inquiry. They discuss the art of crafting questions that "…intrigue, that work the mind, that touch the heart and that render meanings that can orient people … to new possibilities for [sic] change and development by making better use of insider knowledges" (p. 491). Epston, sharing what makes a good question, stresses how they "…have a dramatic effect. They wake you up. They breathe life into you by revitalizing and inspiriting all your senses" (p. 492). I strive to ask questions in this way, which stir interest about the more neglected territories of identity, future prospects for life, or invite deliberation about the significance of one's responses to life difficulties.

Inquiring about "interest" particularly assists my skill development working with youth who may find many more things interesting than a single session conversation. I am challenged to find questions and "ways of not disadvantaging youth" (Bird, 2004) in these conversations. This has led to the exploration of ways to bring poetics into my questions, use of activity, and take-away documents, as ways, as David Epston has said, to "re-energize the narrative" to keep the participants engaged in the conversation.

Your Skills

Of great importance to a brief narrative single session process is the foregrounding of the skills, know-how, and wisdom of the children, youth and adults who consult us. Canvasing what participants bring to the process and working primarily with their know-how fosters the experience of personal agency. It is when the single session becomes instructional or privileging outsider knowledge that I believe SST can become concerning. Building from people's own experiences and what they already know how to do assists the conversation to be contextual, cultural relevant and safer in general.

For this reason, we ask people to discern if the therapist learned about their skills, know-how, and wisdom or did not make that part of the process (Madsen, 2007). Low ratings on this item tells us that we have perhaps become overly instructional. It is a clue informing us that we need to exercise our "double listening" (White, 2003) skills more as well as our inquiry into what people bring to the process and how their knowledge can be used to address their concerns. This measure shapes our practice in orienting us to pay attention to ways that professional knowledge and local knowledge take up space in the conversation.

Partnership

Partnership is an important aspect in our conversations. This refers to facilitating a process in which children and adults experience having a say and playing a part in contributing to the outcome. Attention to this skill pushes me to examine my de-centred influential posture (White & Morgan, 2006), and to scrutinize my ways of creating space for everyone's contribution, including young children. I give attention to practices that don't disadvantage children but rather engage them such as through art or play, or play-acting. I invite people to discern partnership, contrasting the experience of being an important partner in our work together on that day to experiencing being left out of the work (Madsen, 2007). Feedback regarding people's experience of partnership holds me to my relational ethic of striving to level the hierarchy, keeping the participants ideas and input at the centre of the work and sharing in the process.

Feedback

Creating feedback loops throughout the session are especially important in SST as a means to stay relevant and useful to participants. Without future contacts we will not have the chance to check in to see if the therapy is useful and if we have been addressing together what people have come for. As a means to stay aligned with the participants hope for their time with us, periodically throughout the conversation I will ask several questions seeking the persons feedback regarding a) how the conversation is going for them, b) if it has been useful to that point, c) what has or hasn't been useful, d) what stands out for them that we should talk more about, and e) whether I should be asking about a different topic.

Feedback loops provide a means to co-shape the conversation as it unfolds. Similar to tacking in sailing, feedback assists us to monitor and adjust as we go. Eliciting feedback invites accountability to the established project agreed upon at the outset and supports a collaborative process. It is an important skill and I believe contributes to people's sense of feeling heard and understood. I invite people to contrast, "Did your therapist ask for your feedback throughout the conversation" to "My therapist continued without checking in with me" (Duncan et al., 2000).

Next Steps/Plans

A priority in brief narrative work is to facilitate a process in which proposals for action and/or next steps become available for people. As noted in Chapter 7, this is in contrast to practices in which the therapist would provide homework, advice, suggestions, recommendations, or interventions to the participant. My preference is for next steps and plans to come from the people consulting us to guard against offering highly decontextualized ideas that may not be relevant to the person once they return to the context in which they live.

To elicit feedback on co-developing or assisting people to come up with their own ideas, I ask them to distinguish between "I played a large part in developing the plan and next steps" and "I played no part in developing the plan and next steps". Should they score their experience more towards not playing a part in developing the plan or next steps, it serves as an indicator to the therapist about the need for reflection and skill development. The therapist is invited to ask the following questions: What ways could I have invited the participants to come up with their own ideas? What might the possible effects be on their sense of personal agency when only I provide the ideas? What conversation could we have had that would provide for a well of ideas to turn into proposals for action after the session?

Seeking answers to these questions has shaped my practice, having me integrate the consistent use of session re-tellings, and questions that emerge from those re-tellings that assist people to re-contextualize the conversation as discussed in Chapter 7.

Hope

It seems commonsensical that we would want people to leave their session with a sense of hope for the future. Indeed, hope plays a role in contributing to successful therapeutic outcomes (Duncan, Miller, Wampold & Hubble, 2010). In defining "hope" I'm drawn to Snyder's hope equation (see Snyder, 1994). Simply, hope can be seen as a culmination of people's sense that they can do something about their concern (personal agency) and the formation of ideas about what to do about it (options for proceeding or pathways).

Snyder's representation fits well with my intent to facilitate therapeutic conversations that sponsor people's experience of personal agency (I can do something about this) and assist in defining doable next steps (I know what to do). For this reason, I have felt it important to ask after the session about people's sense of hope. Similar to Johnson (1994), I ask them to discern between "I felt hopeful after the session" and "I felt hopeless after the session".

Low scoring on hope cues me in two ways. First, a low rating prompts me to check in with the participants to inquire about their sense of safety and if some safety planning needs to happen. Second, a low rating invites me into reflection about the kinds of questions I could have asked that may have contributed to hope. This, again, is especially important as I do not have the luxury of future sessions to address mishaps. Fine-tuning our hope friendly process is an important project.

I also want to add that a low hope score does not always indicate a concern about the session. In some conversations as people come to revise their position on a problem it makes sense that their hope rating would lower. For instance, someone who arrives and profits from selling drugs who had little concern about these actions may come to see their situation differently in session. They may come to reflect on the consequences of their actions on their relationship with family. They may come to consider harm to others and how they are viewed by members of the community. In review of these circumstances, it can happen that the participants come to new conclusions about selling drugs and the direction of their life. They may struggle to know how to proceed given this new vantage point. This shift would affect their hope for the future even those the revised position itself may be a promising development. Still, in this circumstance it is important to check in regarding personal safety.

Usefulness

Finally, I ask participants to indicate if they found the conversation useful in contrast to not finding it useful. This is an outcome that is important to me and often important to funders, and governing bodies. I do not ask if the conversation was helpful. I prefer to ask if the session was useful as that is congruent with narrative intent. I resist a posture of helping people in favour of striving to be useful to them by facilitating a process. I resist a helping posture as in the context of a single session that posture risks inviting practices that may erode personal agency placing the therapist at the center of change. Further, it may be too soon to tell if the session was helpful for participants. Immediately following the session people will have a sense if the conversation was useful in providing a new or different way of looking at things or ideas for proceeding.

Assisting the Conversation to Endure

Chapter 7 outlines our efforts to assist these conversations to endure long after the face-to-face contact. The last question on the SSIFT provides one last opportunity to elicit and highlight takeaways from the conversation. To facilitate this, I include on the questionnaire the question, "What are one or two things that stood out for you in the conversation that were useful and will stay with you when you leave"? In answering, the participants are generating a specific idea, most relevant to them, for further consideration. The answer gives us a peek into what may stay with them following the conversation. When that is highlighted in combination with receiving a take-away document, the endurance of the conversation is less vulnerable to fatigue.

Closing

This chapter has shared the Single Session Impressions and Feedback Tool (SSIFT)©, a quick access, single session therapy process/outcome feedback tool congruent with the practice intentions of brief narrative therapy. When we link the process (how we do what we do) to the outcome (the usefulness of what we do) in single session therapy our attention becomes focused on the process of therapy and the possible effects of those processes on people's lives. Further, the tool shapes the practices of the therapist inviting critical reflection, accountability and learning. With the proliferation of walk-in clinic service models throughout Canada and abroad the need for tools that provide data for funders, as well as clinicians will continue to grow. The tool presented, although more a part of a "collaborative ethnographic" endeavour, serves to respond to the need for an outcome measure of single session therapy while ensuring a structure and procedure for reflection is in place.

Notes

1 Parts of this chapter were previously published as Cooper, S. Quality assurance at the walk-in clinic: Process outcome and learning [online]. *International Journal of Narrative Therapy & Community Work*, 4(2013), 30–37 and are reshared here with permission.
2 This was informal research grouping the comments provided over five years on the SSIFT at a quick access clinic for children and families. I never had time to formally publish, however as warm data, I believe it starts to paint a useful picture. Process included comments about people's experience of the process, all that happens in the therapy. Actions included comments related to new actions or strategies that people are leaving with to try out to address their circumstances. Resources refers to learning about external service resources that may provide a better fit or timing to assist them to address their circumstances. Thinking refers to people's shifting view of themselves or their situation.

References

Bird, J. (2004). *Talk that sings: Therapy in a new linguistic key*. Auckland: Edge Press.
Catalina, S. (2022). Mental health walk-in clinics for children and families. *Electronic Thesis and Dissertation Repository*, 8613. https://ir.lib.uwo.ca/etd/8613
Children's Mental Health Ontario Position Statement (2013). *Towards a sustainable future: Working together to transform Ontario's child and youth mental health system—part 1*. Retrieved June 2013, www.kidsmentalhealth.ca/documents/res-towards-a-sustainable-future.pdf
Cooper, S. (2013). Quality assurance at the walk-in clinic: Process, outcome, and learning [online]. *International Journal of Narrative Therapy & Community Work*, 4, 30–37.
Duncan, B. (2012). The partners for change outcome management system (PCOMS): The heart and soul of change project. *Canadian Psychology/ Psychologie Canadienne*, *53*, 93–104. http://dx.doi.org/10.1037/ a0027762
Duncan, B. & Miller, S. (2000). *The heroic client: Doing client-directed, outcome informed therapy*. San Francisco: Jossey-Bass.
Duncan, B.L., Miller, S.D. & Sparks, J.A. (2004). *The heroic client: A revolutionary way to improve effectiveness through client-directed, outcome-informed therapy*. San Francisco: Jossey-Bass.
Duncan, B., Miller, S., Wampold, B. & Hubble, M. (Eds.). (2010). *The heart and soul of change: Delivering what works in therapy (2nd ed.)*. Washington, DC: American Psychological Association. http://dx.doi.org/10.1037/12075-000
Hancock, F. & Epston, D. (2008). The craft and art of narrative inquiry in organizations. In D. Barry & H. Jensen (Eds.), *Sage handbook of new approaches in management and organization* (pp. 485–479). London: Sage Publications.

Johnson, L.D. (1995). *Psychotherapy in the age of accountability*. New York: Norton.

Lambert, M. (2010). *Prevention of treatment failure: The use of measuring, monitoring, and feedback in clinical practice*. Washington, DC: American Psychological Association. http://dx.doi.org/10.1037/12141-000

Lassiter, L. E. (2005). *The Chicago guide to collaborative ethnography*. Chicago: The University of Chicago Press.

Madsen, W.C. (2007). Chapter 10: Sustaining collaborative practice in the real world. *Collaborative therapy with multi-stressed families*. New York: Guilford Press.

Miller, S. D., Duncan, B. L., Brown, J., Sparks, J. & Claud, D. (2003). The outcome rating scale: A preliminary study of the reliability, validity, and feasibility of a brief visual analog measure. *Journal of Brief Therapy, 2*, 91–100.

Orlinsky, D. E., Ronnestad, M. H. & Willutzki, U. (2004). Fifty years of psychotherapy process-outcome research: Continuity and change. In M.J. Lambert (Ed.), Bergin and Garfield's *Handbook of psychotherapy and behaviour change* (5th ed., pp. 307–389). New York: Wiley.

Snyder, C. R. (1994). *The psychology of hope*. New York: The Free Press.

Stiles, W. (2002). Session evaluation questionnaire: Structure and use. Retrieved March 2013 from www.users.miamioh.edu/stileswb/session_evaluation_questionnaire.htm

White, M. (2003). Narrative practice and community assignments. *International Journal of Narrative Therapy and Community Work, 2003*(2), 17–55.

White, M. (2007). *Maps of narrative practice*. New York: W.W. Norton.

White, M. (2011). *Narrative practice: Continuing the conversations*. New York: W.W. Norton.

White, M. & Morgan A. (2006). *Narrative therapy with children and their families*. Adelaide. South Australia: Dulwich Centre Publications.

Chapter 19

Conclusion

I was brought up gardening. My parents fostered a garden each summer which led to the annual treat of fresh beans, tomatoes, and Swiss chard. The accompanying smells that went with pickling and making relish can still take me back in time to those warm summer days, grinding cucumbers and making strawberry jam outside on the picnic table. As the years went on my dad grew seedlings. That became a yearly tradition with Grace and Ben helping. We eventually planted our own gardens, not near as big as mom and dads but productive just the same. Brief narrative single session conversations remind a lot of gardening. They are fertile ground for meaning generation, they germinate meaning, and are part of the larger ecology of life.

Nora Bateson, an educator, ecology thinker, and daughter of Gregory Bateson, has used the metaphor of *compost* for describing what goes on in the ecology of communication (Bateson, 2022). Perhaps brief narrative conversations are like meaning making compost. The context provides fertile ground for meanings to emerge, revise, and decompose. Preferred meanings, while conceivably germinated in the moment, unfold over time, may be nourishing or lie dormant until the conditions make sense for new sprouts of understanding to be established. Everything brought to the conversation is part of the process allowing for unexpected connections and emergent offshoots to possibility and difference. I quite like this metaphor.

While my aim in crafting this book has been to provide an orientation to brief narrative single session therapy, I want to stress that the practice will always be incomplete–composting too, germinating, sprouting, and becoming. There will always be more to learn. As mentioned, the context of single session therapy is demanding. Despite this, the therapy is not rushed but rather nuanced requiring a certain mindset and accompanying skills that assist to weave events together, connecting, and exploring meanings ascribed to those events. The brevity is an outcome of the way we see and hear the world, it comes about through attention to the details of the emerging knowledge co-created through engaging conversation.

DOI: 10.4324/9781003431688-20

Periodically I meet service providers who still share a pessimism about the usefulness of narrative practice let alone narrative practice and single session therapy. Skepticism is useful and any therapy practiced should be under a cloud of review and reflection as there is no perfect therapy. Yet, if you believe in people, and can embrace the amazing multiplicities of meaning making, the plurality of any expression, the potential of these conversations is revealed. It takes hard work though, and a great deal of practice. Drift too is inevitable as we are surrounded by the discourses of the day; some extremely influential in shaping our mindset and trying to calibrate our ear. For this reason, regular review, check-ins along the way, and meaningful supervision make a difference and are important. Attention to relational ethics will serve this process well, assisting us to craft a just practice.

The ideas in this book hopefully provide a foundation upon which you can craft your own voice, style, and brief narrative practice. Make it your own, add what you can to your current awesomeness and feel welcome to leave behind what doesn't yet fit. I hope the field can stay inspired by the spirit of exploration and discovery set forth by those practitioners and teachers that have shaped the contemporary brief therapies.

One last question: when is your book coming out? The field will benefit from your experiences, and I invite you to write and share, as Yvonne Dolan did with me that day back in 2001.

Reference

Bateson, N. (2022). New words to hold the invisible world of possibility part 3: apha-nipoiesis. *Unpsychology*. Retrieved July 29, 2023, from https://unpsychology.subst ack.com/p/new-words-to-hold-the-invisible-world-d90.

Appendix 1

Drop-In Therapy Clinic Participant Questionnaire, Parent/Guardian

This appendix provides an example of the single session therapy pre-session questionnaire for parent and guardians. Also see Young et al., 2008 for other possibilities.

Company Logo   **DROP-IN THERAPY CLINIC PARTICIPANT QUESTIONNAIRE** *PARENT/GUARDIAN*

Child/Youth Name:		Today's Date:	
Birth Gender:	Identifies As:	Date of Birth (mm,dd,yyyy):	Age:
Address:	Street Address:	City: Postal Code:	
Phone (H):		School: Grade:	
Phone (Cell):		Family Doctor:	
Permission To: *Call Leave Message Text* ☐ ☐ ☐		Parent/Legal Guardian:	
Email:		Lives With: Phone #:	

Family Members:

Given Name	Surname	Birth Date	Relationship	Birth Gender	In Home Yes / No	Age	Attending Session

List any other services you are involved in:	
How did you hear about this clinic?	
Have you been to or contacted the Crisis Service before? Yes ☐ No ☐	Are you, your child, or anyone with you, at risk of harm to self or to others? Yes ☐ No ☐ Who?

I/We understand this organization does not provide opinions or recommendations for the purpose of custody/access matters: ☐	Are you currently involved in any legal process regarding custody & access? Yes ☐ No ☐
Financial stress: Yes ☐ No ☐	

1. What concerns have brought you here today?

   _____

   _____

2. If 10 is the most and 1 is the least, how concerned are you about this?

   Not Really   1   2   3   4   5   6   7   8   9   10   Very

3. What would be important for us to know about the background of this concern?

   _____

   _____

4. What would be most useful to talk about in this meeting today?

   _____

   _____

5. What would someone else come to admire and respect most about your child if they had months or years to get to know them? It's OK to guess.

   _____

   _____

6. For us to be most useful, is there anything important for us to know about your child's culture, ethnicity, religion, language, sexual orientation, gender identity/expression, mental or physical health, or other?

_____

_____

7. With 10 being the best and 1 is very poor, please rate your child's quality of sleep:

Very Poor   1   2   3   4   5   6   7   8   9   10   Best

Appendix 2

Drop-In Therapy Clinic Participant Questionnaire, Child/Youth

This appendix provides an example of the single session therapy pre-session questionnaire for youth. Also see Young et al., 2008 for other possibilities.

Agency Logo   **DROP-IN THERAPY CLINIC**
                    PARTICIPANT QUESTIONNAIRE
                    CHILD/YOUTH

Birth Name:			Today's Date:	
Birth Gender:	I Identify As:	Pronouns:	Date of Birth (mm,dd,yyyy):	Age:
Address:	Street Address:	City:		Postal Code:
Phone (H):			School: Grade:	
Phone (Cell):			Family Doctor:	
Permission To: *Call* *Leave Message* *Text* ☐ ☐ ☐			Parent/Legal Guardian:	
Email:			Parent/Legal Guadian Phone #:	

1. What would someone else like and respect most about you if they had a lot of time to get to know you? It's okay to guess!

_____

_____

_____

2. What would be most important for us to talk about today?

_____

_____

_____

3. When are things better – even a little bit?

_____

_____

_____

4. If 10 is the best and 1 is the worst, how are things in your life today?

   Worst   1   2   3   4   5   6   7   8   9   10   Best

5. With 10 being the best and 1 is very poor, how would you rate your quality of sleep?

   Very Poor   1   2   3   4   5   6   7   8   9   10   Best

6. Are you currently at risk of harm to yourself or to others? Yes ☐ No ☐

7. For us to be most useful, is there anything important for us to know about your culture, ethnicity, spirituality, language, sexual orientation, gender identity/expression, mental or physical health, or other?

   _____

   _____

   _____

Appendix 3

Conversation Summary

This conversation summary was inspired by Kormans' (2005) Magic Square and adapted for brief narrative single session therapy. It's typically a double sided document. Originally it served as a teaching tool. If the problem quadrant had filled up it was a visual signal to the therapist to ask other kinds of questions to get on to difference. However, as participants found it useful to have a copy, it became a popular take away document as a Conversation Summary.

Conversation Summary Single Session Therapy Clinic	Name:		Date:	
	DOB:		Age:	
Therapist Name(s):				
☐ No Identified Risk	☐ Risk/Safety Addressed		Consent Signed	☐
			Consent Verbal	☐

SAFETY STEPS

\
\
\
\
\
\
\
\
\
\
\
\
\
\
\
\
\
\

_____   _____

Lead Therapist Signature   *Date*

_____   _____

2nd Therapist Signature   *Date*

BACKGROUND / INTERESTS / SKILLS / ABILITIES	HOPES FOR TODAY
	PROBLEM / CONCERN
INITIATIVES	PRACTICE PLAN / NEXT STEPS

HOPES FOR TODAY

- What would be most important for us to talk about today?
- How might you know this time is useful to you when you leave?
- What would your best friend say needs to happen here for this to be useful?

PROBLEM / CONCERN

- **Questions to elicit and honour the concern.**
  - What would be most important for us to talk about today given we have this one time together?
  - How can this conversation be useful to you?
  - What kinds of things have you tried to date?
  - Externalizing practices.
  - Who, what, where, when of the problem.
- **Contexting:**
  - What's the history of the problem/concern in your life?
  - What is it in relation to? Discourses? How does it make sense given what people have experienced?

BACKGROUND / INTERESTS / SKILLS / ABILITIES

- **Questions to meet through stories of competence.**
  - What is it you have come to know and appreciate about your child that lives outside the problem description?
  - What is it you tell your friends that you love about your child, that you brag about to them?
  - What are your interests, what are you in to?
  - What are you passionate about?
- **Questions that invite the introduction of other people in their life, significant relationships.**
  - Who is your best friend?
  - What are your partners' ideas about this concern?
  - Re-membering conversations.
- **Non-structural accounts of life**
  - Intentions for life, values, beliefs about how things should be.
  - Commitments, moral codes, hopes, wishes, preferences, etc.
  - What are your ideas about how people should be in relationships?

INITIATIVES	PRACTICE PLAN / NEXT STEPS

• **Questions to inquire about times when the problem was not around or less, counter thoughts, feelings, actions.**
 • Externalizing Conversations Map #2.
 • Tell me about the times when this problem was not as bad?
 • Point of reference questions.
   — If 10 is on track and 1 the opposite, where would you say things are now?
   — What would a small step (from 3 to 3.5) look like?
 • Initiative questions.
   — When don't you, or didn't you have this problem?
   — What is different at those times?
 • **Begin linking and naming.**
   — What would you call what you did if you were to give it thought?
   — What would you call these things you have done and thought?
   — Is that like confidence, using bravery, using pretending, wisdom, perseverance?
   — Is this a "plan", "strategy", "proposal"?
	• **Questions to discern next steps, practice areas, and action plans.**
	   — Given that we talked about ....what ideas are coming to mind about the next step you will take when you leave here today?
	   — Given our conversation, what will you practice when you leave here that will start the ball rolling?
	   — What might be possible to do that would be more in harmony with what you value, what you are learning that's important to you?
	 • **Questions to begin to address receiving context–Speculating, audiencing, identifying constraints.**
	   — What difference will that make when you leave here?
	   — How long do you suppose you'll need to practice that?
	   — Who will it be essential to share this conversation with?
	   — How will you use this conversation summary?
	   — What may try to get in the way of your practice?
	   — What might happen that tries to take you backwards or off-track?
	   — How will you handle that hurdle, pothole, step back?

Appendix 4

Single Session Impressions and Feedback Tool (SSIFT)©

Name _____ Date _____

Please share your feedback. Please circle the appropriate number to indicate your experience of today's conversation.

Agree with this side	Neutral	Agree with this side

FOCUS
My therapist focused on what they wanted to and my wishes didn't seem important

My therapist addressed what I/we wanted to talk about the most

          1   2   3   4   5   6   7

INTEREST
The conversation was uninteresting to me

The conversation captured and held my interest

          1   2   3   4   5   6   7

YOUR SKILLS
My therapist did not learn about my skills, abilities, or wisdom

My therapist learned about my skills, abilities, and wisdom

          1   2   3   4   5   6   7

PARTNERSHIP
I felt left out of the work today

I experienced being an important partner in our work together today

          1   2   3   4   5   6   7

Agree with this side			Neutral			Agree with this side
FEEDBACK My therapist kept going without checking in with me						My therapist asked for my feedback throughout the conversation
	1	2	3	4	5	6	7
PLANS/NEXT STEPS I played no part in developing the plan and next steps						I played a large part in developing the plan and next steps
	1	2	3	4	5	6	7
HOPE I felt hopeless after the conversation						I felt hopeful after the conversation
	1	2	3	4	5	6	7

What are one or two things that stood out for you in the conversation that were useful and will stay with you when you leave?

1. _____

2. _____

3. _____

Adapted from Lynn Johnson, 1995; Duncan & Miller, 2000; Stiles, 2002; and Madsen, 2007.

Index

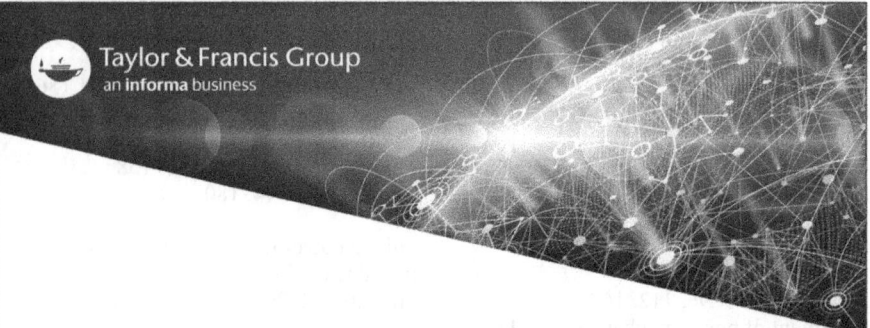
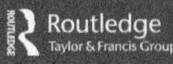
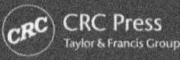